Interventions for Reading Problems

The Guilford Practical Intervention in the Schools Series

Kenneth W. Merrell, Series Editor

Interventions for Reading Problems

Designing and Evaluating Effective Strategies

EDWARD J. DALY III
SANDRA CHAFOULEAS
CHRISTOPHER H. SKINNER

THE GUILFORD PRESS
New York   London

© 2005 The Guilford Press
A Division of Guilford Publications, Inc.
72 Spring Street, New York, NY 10012
www.guilford.com

Printed in Canada

This book is printed on acid-free paper.

Last digit is print number: 9   8   7   6   5   4   3   2   1

Library of Congress Cataloging-in-Publication Data

Daly, Edward J., 1963–
  Interventions for reading problems: designing and evaluating effective strategies / Edward J. Daly III, Sandra Chafouleas, Christopher H. Skinner.
      p. cm. — (Guilford practical intervention in the schools series)
  Includes bibliographical references and index.
  ISBN 1-59385-081-6 (pbk.: alk. paper)
  1. Reading—Remedial teaching. I. Chafouleas, Sandra. II. Skinner, Christopher H.
III. Title. IV. Series.
  LB1050.5.D28 2005
    372.43—dc22
                                                                      2004016665

About the Authors

Edward J. Daly III, PhD, is Associate Professor of Educational (School) Psychology at the University of Nebraska–Lincoln and Program Director of the School Psychology program. Dr. Daly received his doctorate from Syracuse University in 1992 and worked for several years as a school psychologist before becoming a trainer of school psychologists in 1995. His research interests include the application of principles of behavior analysis to resolving children's reading problems. He is especially interested in developing usable and useful technologies for assessing and intervening with children who display reading deficits. Dr. Daly has published numerous articles, books, and book chapters in the fields of school psychology and applied behavior analysis. He served previously as Associate Editor of *School Psychology Review* and *School Psychology Quarterly*, and currently serves as guest action editor and reviewer for a number of professional journals.

Sandra Chafouleas, PhD, is currently Assistant Professor in the School Psychology program at the University of Connecticut. Previously, Dr. Chafouleas directed the School Psychology program at Plattsburgh State University of New York. In both positions, she has provided training in behavioral assessment and intervention to future and practicing school psychologists. She also has taught courses in academic and intellectual assessment, ethics, and the roles and functions of school psychologists. Dr. Chafouleas currently serves on the editorial boards of *School Psychology Review, School Psychology Quarterly*, and *Psychology in the Schools*. Her primary areas of research interest involve the prevention of reading difficulties and the application of evidence-based strategies to the classroom. Prior to becoming a university trainer, Dr. Chafouleas worked as a school psychologist and school administrator in a variety of settings dealing with children with behavior disorders.

Christopher H. Skinner, PhD, received his doctorate in school psychology from Lehigh University in 1989. He is a Fellow of the American Psychological Association and received the Lightner Witmer Award in 1995 for outstanding scholarship from a young academic or professional. Dr. Skinner is coeditor of the *Journal of Behavioral Education.* His research interests include academic interventions, learning and skill development, behavioral and curriculum-based assessment, and single-subject research methodologies. As a behavioral school psychologist, Dr. Skinner's work reflects a commitment to advancing the science of school psychology through applied and theoretical research. As a former special education teacher, his research also focuses on applied procedures that can be used to prevent and remedy student problems. Currently he serves as coordinator of School Psychology Programs at the University of Tennessee.

Acknowledgments

We would like to thank our spouses (Amy, Anne, and E. J.) for their support through this project. We are grateful to Jim Wright for his great (and tireless) work in disseminating information to practitioners, his willingness to let us use his materials, and also his helpful feedback on drafts of the book. We thank Jenny Burt, who also provided insightful feedback on drafts of the book. We express sincere appreciation for our wonderful mentors, who have taught us so much over the years and who continue to inspire us: Ed Lentz, Larry Lewandowski, Brian Martens, Ed Shapiro, and Joe Witt. Finally, Edward J. Daly wishes to thank, above all, Him "through whom I can do all things" (Philippians 4:13).

Contents

List of Tables, Figures,
and Worksheets

TABLES

FIGURES

WORKSHEETS

1

Introduction and Overview

Just think for a moment about what you are doing right now and about how often throughout the day (*each* and *every* day) you rely on the very skill you are applying to this text. For those of us fortunate enough to learn this vital skill, we do it so often we barely think about how it impacts our lives. The Greek philosopher Aristotle stated that we don't need to know we have a brain to think. Likewise, a proficient reader doesn't need to know, or be conscious of, the processes that allow reading to happen. Some of you may even be "multitasking" right now—which only proves our point. More likely, someone else thought about and planned relevant reading experiences for us so that it would become automatic. We may take for granted the many complex experiences that had to be planned for us to become facile readers. Table 1.1 highlights some of the most critical accomplishments necessary to make reading a useful activity for learning and enjoyment.

TABLE 1.1. Reading Encompasses a Wide Variety of Skills

- The skills and knowledge to understand how speech sounds are related to print
- The ability to decode or decipher unfamiliar words
- The ability to read fluidly and quickly
- Sufficient background information and vocabulary to foster understanding
- The development of strategies to extract the meaning of the text
- Motivation to read

Note. From U.S. Department of Education (1999).

1

Staggering numbers of students have difficulty with reading. Based on data from 2002 assessments, the National Center for Educational Statistics (NCES, 2003) reported that only a third of 4th, 8th, and 12th graders read at or above the "proficient" level. Two-thirds of 4th graders and only three-fourths of 8th and 12th graders read at or above the "basic" level. The stability of the results across grade levels is remarkable. If we project these results across grade levels, they suggest that approximately 23 million children of school age have not attained proficiency in reading (based on the estimated 70 million children in the United States; NCES, 2003). The problem is so great that the No Child Left Behind Act established a federally funded national initiative—Reading First—to improve reading instruction in kindergarten through third-grade classrooms (U.S. Department of Education, 2004). Reading First is a $900 million state grant program that will help states and local school districts adopt and implement scientifically based methods of reading instruction. Reading is obviously foundational to most other subjects that students study in school and to most activities after graduation. Reading problems can have an extremely adverse effect on quality of life, limiting educational and employment opportunities as well as access to a variety of enjoyable activities.

Unfortunately, schools generally have not been sufficiently organized to meet the needs of students who have reading problems or students who came to school ill prepared to learn to read. Preservice teachers take, on average, 1.3 courses in reading instruction in university training programs, and most basal reading series are inadequate for guiding teachers in teaching reading to a diverse student body (National Research Council, 1998). Those with expertise in assessment and consultation are often called upon to help in cases where children are having difficulty learning to read. In some instances, however, these professionals may be even less prepared to resolve reading difficulties than the teachers and administrators who turn to them. This book takes the perspective of the consultant who is working with others to solve a problem, regardless of whether it is an individual child problem (e.g., a fourth grader referred for reading problems) or a systemwide problem (e.g., a large number of students with low reading levels in a school). That said, we hope that this book will be useful to teachers too. Reflective teachers consult with themselves (hopefully, not aloud!) and often engage in problem solving by themselves or with colleagues.

The purpose of this book is to provide a comprehensive but concise overview of how to improve reading performance for children who are having difficulty learning to read. The book has a procedural or "how-to" focus and describes how to assess and intervene with reading problems and evaluate outcomes of interventions. It addresses the full range of reading problems, from early literacy, when students are establishing the building blocks for successful reading, to complex comprehension problems that may manifest themselves in content areas such as science or social studies. In addition to addressing assessment and intervention for students who already exhibit reading problems, a portion of the book is devoted to examining reading difficulties from a broader, systems-level perspective. In some school districts the sheer number of children with reading problems challenges educators to find and implement efficient prevention and remediation strategies. We hope that the up-to-date content for best practices across the spectrum of reading needs and the descriptions of methods for choosing and evaluating interventions will serve you well in your practice. The strategies we offer are scientifically based. More importantly, however, you will be given methods for investigating, yourself, whether those scientifically based strategies are working for your students—the real essence of science-based practice. You might be confident that a proven method will work, but you won't really know until you try it out with the student(s). This process is one of validating an already scientifically valid method for a particular student or group of students. You might think of it as *local validation*, a type of mini-scientific experiment with the student(s) with whom you are working.

CHARACTERISTICS OF THE APPROACH TAKEN IN THIS BOOK

It all starts with getting the wrong answer. A parent is reviewing letters with her child, for example, and he says *b* for *p*. A teacher points to the word *cat* and the student says *cab*. A teacher notices that the student didn't answer the independent seatwork questions correctly. There's a problem. Maybe the child simply didn't understand. The parent says, "Let's try again. What is this letter?" If the child gets it right the second time around, the adult moves on and may not think about it any further. However, if the child gets it wrong the second time, the parent or teacher corrects the child ("No. That's a *b*. Can you say *b*?") and makes a mental note. If it happens often enough—if the child eventually gives one wrong answer too many—the adult will realize that there is a problem. On the other hand, as long as the child is giving the right answer, there is no need to infer a problem. Indeed, our natural tendency is to assume the contrary. We come to believe that he or she "knows" or "has learned" and we are satisfied with the child's performance as long as the answers are correct.

The point of departure for the task at hand is when the child gives one-too-many wrong answers. Therefore, this book is not intended to focus primarily on reading instruction (although designing reading interventions requires knowing something about effective reading instruction) or structuring curricula (although designing reading interventions often requires modifications to curricular materials and how instruction is delivered). Rather, it is all about problem solving when one or more students are not giving right answers during the course of typical instruction in the curriculum. The regular curriculum (and all the other experiences in and out of school) may be fine for the majority of students. The focus here is on those students who are perceived by teachers, parents, or others as having a problem.

We take a *functional* approach in this book, as noted in Table 1.2. First, we evaluate a child's ability to read by having him or her read and not by giving complicated tests to make sophisticated diagnoses. In other words, we advocate for assessing student performance directly in the curriculum. Not only has this proven to be the best method for addressing reading problems, but it also increases clarity of communication with stakeholders. We aren't talking about concepts that only the most sophisticated measurement

TABLE 1.2. Characteristics of a Functional Approach to Reading Intervention

1. Student performance is assessed directly in the curriculum.
2. Intervention targets student performance in important curricular tasks.
3. The intervention is focused on the components of instruction and the procedures necessary to improve ongoing instruction.
4. Observable and measurable improvement in student learning, over time, is the criterion for successful intervention.

person can understand. With a complete and adequate explanation, most constituents (parents, teachers, and others) can understand the importance of reading assessment measures such as correctly read words per minute and errors per minute (methods explained in later chapters). In fact, when assessment data are plotted on a graph, our constituents can decide *for themselves* whether the outcomes were positive or not. They no longer need to rely on the expert to interpret results for them. Instead, *they* are empowered to address their children's or students' needs better (Erchul & Martens, 2002). The overall outcome is likely to be more positive for the children.

Furthermore, because the focus of our attention is on how well the child reads in the classroom or home context, the goal of intervention is to assist the child to read and react appropriately to the content in ways that teachers and parents expect (e.g., through answering comprehension questions). If an intervention is successful, the child is now answering correctly (thereby reversing the trajectory of wrong answers that led the teacher or parent to perceive a problem in the first place). This approach to intervention is a direct one, in which assistance to the learner facilitates frequent, correct answers. Viewed in this way, the goal of reading intervention is deceptively simple: We strive to do what it takes to help students "get it right" when the teacher or parent wants an answer. In Chapter 2, we discuss a learning model—the instructional hierarchy—that helps you understand how to achieve this goal. Chapters 3, 4, and 5 describe techniques that address early reading, fluency, and comprehension problems, respectively. The instructional hierarchy model explains why the interventions work and when a particular intervention strategy is appropriate; the model therefore serves as the overarching framework for the intervention process.

Intervention involves primarily having the student read a lot and using methods that facilitate correct answers. Because we have defined the task as a problem-solving one we emphasize the *components* of instruction more than general reading curricula or instruction from start to finish. Our assumption is that some type of reading instruction is being delivered but is not helping students to get right answers. As noted earlier, it is the preponderance of wrong answers that leads to the realization of a problem. We don't expect, however, that you are in a position to radically alter the curriculum that is being presented to the student. Consultants rarely are in this position when they are taking a case-centered approach to intervention. We are not referring to, or even addressing, curriculum consultants who may be called in to help a school district evaluate various reading curricula. Instead, it may be the special educator, the school psychologist, or the external consultant who is called upon to conduct assessments and provide recommendations for one or more children. In this case, the best approach is to analyze the components of instruction (and instructional tasks) to determine what is missing so that the evaluator can assist teachers in making current instruction more effective. Therefore, in most cases teachers won't be expected to stop and start all over again. Interventions that target adjustments and modifications to ongoing classroom routines and instruction will probably be more successful than interventions that involve changing everything the teacher is currently doing. A major task of diagnosing the learner is diagnosing the instruction the learner is receiving (Engelmann, Granzin, & Severson, 1979). As this book outlines the components of instruction that facilitate better reading, specific attention is paid to the procedures that should be followed to improve student reading. When possible, we have included step-by-step protocols for a number of different types of interventions.

To illustrate this approach, we turn to a recently published study that targeted remediation of severe reading problems related to accuracy and fluency. In an effort to remediate severe reading problems, Torgesen et al. (2001) provided instruction to 60 students with severe reading problems on a one-to-one basis two times a week for 50 minutes per session over a period of 8–9 weeks. The instructional intervention was explicit and systematic. Activities targeting accuracy and fluency skill building in phonemic awareness and individual word reading and writing were delivered using one of two approaches: auditory discrimination or phonics. Following accuracy and fluency building, generalization training (i.e., practice applying the skills in the classroom) occurred once per week for an additional 8 weeks. Student progress on multiple outcome measures was tracked for 2 years. Results suggested that both programs were equally effective in producing substantial improvement over the long term. In fact, over half of the students demonstrated accelerated reading growth to an extent that allowed them to fall within the normal range. This finding is amazing, given the severity of the deficits exhibited by the students prior to receiving the intervention. Thus, overall results suggested that the specific instructional activities were not as important as the inclusion of components of instruction that systematically built accuracy and fluency and then taught students to generalize newly learned skills to classroom curricular tasks. In this study, these principles included explicit instruction involving direct teaching and modeling along with multiple opportunities to practice and receive feedback.

Although the participants in this study were older children who already exhibited significant reading problems and the interventions were more intensive than is instruction typically available in the school setting, implications can be drawn regarding effective reading instruction for all students. Torgesen et al. (2001) suggested that two factors were important in producing substantial growth over the long term: the right level of intensity and teacher skill. In other words, the teacher must have the skill to assess an individual student's instructional needs, choose instructional strategies targeting those needs, and then monitor the effects of instruction. Students with reading problems require explicit and systematic instruction that is matched to their skill level. Effective instruction provides ample opportunity for guided practice with new concepts and cues students when to use skills in classroom activities. The conclusion? There is probably more than one way to go about teaching basic reading skills, but certain factors, such as explicit and systematic instruction and progress monitoring (among others), are minimally necessary to get the job done.

Professionals have an ethical and a legal responsibility to be accountable for student outcomes, lest students be deprived of their right to a *free and appropriate education* (Jacob & Hartshorne, 2003). This responsibility means that we must evaluate whether students are learning. Otherwise, we can't call what's being done *instruction*. It amounts to nothing more than presenting the curriculum. The best way to measure learning is to systematically examine student progress over time—that is, the process of local validation to which we referred earlier. If a referred student is behind others, he or she needs to catch up and attain at least the minimal skills necessary to be successful in other parts of the curriculum. Not only is *rate of learning over time* the single best indicator of improvement, it also tells educators the degree to which students are catching up with their classmates. For these reasons, *observable and measurable improvement in student learning over time* is *the* criterion for successful intervention and constitutes the core principle of science-based practice. In order to accelerate student performance, interventions (and not just students) are evaluated and modified based on assessments over time.

BRIEF OVERVIEW OF THE BOOK

The first objective of this book is to create a context for consulting and conducting reading interventions. Knowing procedures for improving reading will only get you so far if you don't understand the developmental process of acquiring reading and what effective teaching looks like. Also, you need to understand the dynamics of how to facilitate reading interventions if you are not the one actually carrying out the intervention. Each of these issues is discussed in Chapter 2. The next three chapters (3, 4, and 5) address the three broad areas identified by the research literature as comprising the process of reading development: "alphabetics," oral reading fluency, and comprehension. Each chapter begins with a brief rationale for why the skills associated with that domain are critical to becoming a competent reader. Each chapter also gives specific information about assessment and intervention methods. As noted earlier, protocols that outline procedural steps and tables with relevant information about which decisions to make are provided, when needed. Chapter 6, the final chapter, explains various methods for demonstrating results. This step is especially important if you are trying to justify the value of a reading program in the eyes of professionals, authorities, and other constituents. This chapter goes beyond describing individual results and shows how to demonstrate effectiveness (or, if you are less successful, areas where change is needed) across students. This step may be the most important part of the process for evaluating the integrity of your intervention model, if you plan to do more than just a single intervention.

In summary, this book provides a full-service guide to directly assessing, consulting about, and developing reading interventions when there is classroom instruction of some type already in place. Simple and effective instructional strategies for the target areas of alphabetics, fluency, and comprehension are included. Finally, a model for evaluation of effectiveness across cases is included to help you demonstrate accountability for your services. It is our hope that you will find this information useful in your daily efforts to help children become successful readers.

2

Where Do You Start as a Consultant?

Although your eyes are probably riveted to the child referred for reading problems, we invite you to change your focus momentarily to understand more broadly why the child is having a problem with reading tasks in the first place. Diagnosing the child with tests will not be very fruitful if you fail to consider the impact of the classroom and instruction on the student's performance. Engelmann, Granzin, and Severson (1979) put it bluntly when they pointed out that "the only way to draw conclusions about deficiencies involves first determining the degree to which the learner's performance is controlled by instruction" (p. 362). It is critical, therefore, to first diagnose the instruction the child is receiving. You need not take your eyes off the child, however. We suggest instead a broader visual field, which means that you may need to step back. Within this broader field, your focus will shift periodically from the child to other factors and back to the child. The child should *never* leave your field of vision entirely.

This chapter addresses effective reading instruction by focusing on critical attributes of effective reading instruction for students who are at-risk of or currently experiencing reading failure. It differs from the rest of the book in that it describes what could or should be happening *before* a referral. In the following chapters, we emphasize procedures, techniques, and decision steps for intervening once the problem has been detected and one or more students have been referred. The information presented in this chapter, however, is critical to the goals of the latter chapters. As a consultant, you need a template for effective instruction in order to understand the child's problem. This template should guide you in filtering out what is helping the referred student to learn, what is potentially harmful to this learning, and what is missing instructionally.

We begin by discussing the "targets" for reading across the curriculum: various skills in "alphabetics," reading fluency, and comprehension. The targets are the skills children need to master to become proficient readers. These targets serve as prerequisites for more complex skills. (Teachers should organize their instruction around one or more of these targets at any given time.) The delivery of effective instruction is then described, with special emphasis on how instruction should be adapted to the student's level of proficiency. Our goal is to give you a framework for identifying the components of effective reading instruction.

Next we address factors that are likely to impact your ability to effect change as a consultant within the overall organizational school system: the organizational capacity of the school to accept intervention. Failure to acknowledge the school's organizational capacity or incapacity for change may doom the whole enterprise. Finally, the chapter ends with a brief overview of resources available on the Internet. These resources can assist you with the assessment and intervention activities described in the remainder of the book. Consider this chapter as a point of departure for understanding why the child with a reading problem is not progressing successfully and for identifying resources that may be helpful to you in developing reading interventions. The latter chapters on individualized assessment and intervention for early literacy, reading fluency, and reading comprehension have more of a "how-to" focus.

READING TARGETS ACROSS THE CONTINUUM OF READING PROFICIENCY

For students to learn, the teacher must effectively coordinate what is taught, how students are managed during instructional time, and how instruction is delivered in the classroom. Although the process is complex, learning is likely to occur if the student consistently and frequently produces correct responses to reading material in carefully chosen and sequenced instructional activities. How students *respond* is a key element in designing instruction. Consensus has been achieved in the field of reading research regarding the *types of responses* teachers should be teaching. The most prominent example of this consensus can be found in the National Reading Panel (NRP) report (2000). Following a congressional mandate, the NRP reported a synthesis and evaluation of research on reading instruction. The entire report is organized around targets (our term) for instruction. These targets, which include alphabetics, reading fluency, and reading comprehension, have emerged from many years of research reports and other reviews, including but not limited to the report of the National Research Council (NRC, 1998) and the seminal review and summary of Marilyn Adams (1990). Before we explore how teachers manage instruction, we examine each distinct area of reading. Keep in mind that, whereas specific intervention procedures are covered in later chapters, the goal of this chapter is to give you a general understanding of what and how teachers should be teaching so that you can function as a more informed consultant.

Alphabetics refers to the student's ability to manipulate sounds in words ("phonemic awareness") and the acquisition and use of letter–sound correspondences in reading and spelling (phonics; National Reading Panel, 2000). Instruction in phonemic awareness and phonics, the two areas that represent the broader category of alphabetics, helps students to achieve proficiency with these skills. The manipulation of sounds in words requires the ability to isolate sounds in words, delete sounds from words, break words into individual sounds, match sounds, categorize sounds, and blend sounds—all skills that are predictive of reading acquisition (National Reading Panel, 2000). Furthermore, sounds must be linked to letters, the objective of phonics instruction. Different approaches to phonics instruction vary in the degree to which they make the correspondences between letters, sounds, and spelling patterns explicit for students. These correspondences, however, are not useful to students if they are unable to blend sounds together to decode or break them apart to write words (National Reading Panel, 2000). Students need to master both phonemic awareness and phonics. When instruction is successful in teaching these skills, students are able to decode words accurately, which (as the NRP report points out) facilitates comprehension.

Reading fluency refers to accurate, fluid decoding and word recognition. To achieve fluency, a student must read at the appropriate speed. The NRP report describes fluency as "one of several critical factors for reading comprehension" (p. 7) and characterizes the frequent neglect of reading fluency instruction as "unfortunate" (p. 7). Reading fluency is a prerequisite to independent comprehension of text. Anyone who has listened to a child laboriously decode words or text at a rate of one word per 3 seconds (which amounts to a rate of 20 words per minute) understands what it does to the child's ability to understand what he or she is reading. Reading fluency has begun to gain a lot of credibility as a target for assessment and instruction (Chard, Vaughn, & Tyler, 2002; Fuchs, Fuchs, Hosp, & Jenkins, 2001; Kame'enui & Simmons, 2001), thanks to a perceived need for direct and sensitive measures of student performance. Indeed, reading fluency is the single-best indicator of reading proficiency for younger students (Shinn, Good, Knutson, & Tilly, 1992).

Defined as the "essence of reading" by the NRP, the report describes comprehension as a complex cognitive activity that involves intentional problem-solving thinking processes. The panel states: "The data suggest that text comprehension is enhanced when readers actively relate the ideas represented in print to their own knowledge and experiences and construct mental representations in memory" (p. 11). The very complexity of text comprehension requires the teacher to use a combination of instructional techniques to teach effectively. Table 2.1 contains specific instructional strategies recommended by the report for each of the three areas. Although alphabetics and reading fluency are prerequisites to independent text comprehension, the report recommends integration across all three areas—alphabetics, fluency, and comprehension—to create a complete reading program. However, a classroom that neglects the prerequisites and emphasizes a more complex skill (e.g., reading passages aloud) when students are not adept at prior skills (e.g., blending and segmenting sounds) is not meeting the students' needs and (1) makes the learning task more difficult than necessary and (2) slows down the students' progress. As an aside, these circumstances may make the conditions particularly ripe for misbehavior, which is often motivated by a need to escape difficult task demands.

TABLE 2.1. Instructional Strategies Identified by the National Reading Panel (2000) Report for Each Instructional Target

Reading targets	Necessary prerequisite skills	Instruction
Alphabetics		Phonemic awareness and phonics instruction
Reading fluency	Ability to segment and blend words in sounds	Guided, repeated oral reading
Comprehension	Fluent decoding and word recognition	Vocabulary instruction; comprehension monitoring; cooperative learning; use of graphic and semantic organizers (including story maps); question answering and immediate feedback; student-generated questions; use of story structure to help recall of story content; summarization

QUALITIES AND CHARACTERISTICS OF EFFECTIVE READING INSTRUCTION

In the spirit of creating a template for effective instruction, we examine the critical attributes of effective instruction from the perspective of the child who is at risk for, or already experiencing, reading failure. Consistent with effective instructional practices with these students (Lane, Gresham, & O'Shaughnessy, 2002), the approach outlined here involves more explicit forms of teaching. By *explicit* we mean clearer identification of skills and "hands-on" direct instruction that lead the student to mastery (Howell & Kelley, 2002). First, let's imagine that you are walking into the classroom while reading instruction is ongoing. Of course, you have to stay for a while or make several visits to get a complete perspective of how the teacher is instructing. What do you see? Are students working on tasks that are important and helping them to become better readers? Are the lessons and the teacher's interactions with students helping them to read better?

The Instructional Hierarchy

We begin the analysis with the needs of the student. To be effective, instruction must be aligned with each student's level of proficiency. The instructional hierarchy (IH; Haring, Lovitt, Eaton, & Hansen, 1978) is a simple model that has proven useful for understanding why, and under which conditions, instructional procedures are effective (Daly, Lentz, & Boyer, 1996). The basis of this model is a learning hierarchy through which the student progresses as he or she learns a new skill (see Figure 2.1). First, students acquire new responses. At the *acquisition* stage, the new responses are not in the students' repertoire. Therefore, teacher efforts must be directed toward increasing accurate responses and decreasing inaccurate responses. Assuming that students are progressing as expected—that is, they are accurate most of the time and have few errors—the next level of proficiency to achieve is that of fluency. At the *fluency* stage, students respond both accurately and quickly. Fluency is especially critical for reading because readers must quickly and

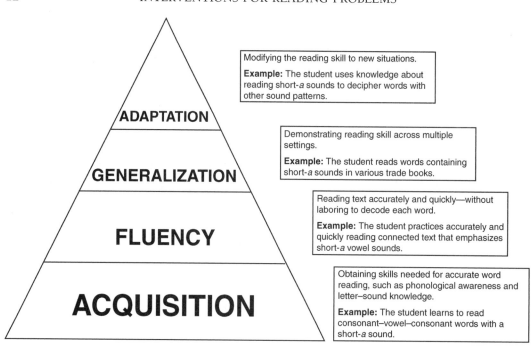

FIGURE 2.1. The instructional hierarchy.

effortlessly identify sequences of letters as words. At this point, teaching strategies should differ from instruction designed to promote acquisition. As we noted earlier, a breakdown in fluency translates into a breakdown in comprehension. Fluency is a necessary but not sufficient condition for overall reading competence. Fluency, as discussed here, is not just oral reading fluency. Students should display fluency in all of the critical targets—alphabetics, phonics, and comprehension—as well as oral reading.

Fluency is not the end goal. The student must be able to generalize the newly fluent skills to new texts, across time, and to more complex skills such as comprehension. The teacher engages in other instructional activities to promote *generalization*. We hesitate to characterize generalization as a next step in a hierarchy for fear that we lead you to believe that the teacher must wait until the student is both accurate and fluent before teaching generalization. Although the strategies that promote generalization differ from those used to promote accuracy and fluency, these strategies should be used throughout the whole instructional process. For example, if the teacher is using flashcards to teach students to read words that appear with high frequency in text (e.g., *the, for, there*), the teacher also should be teaching students to read those words in connected text. Fluency with flashcards does not guarantee that students will be able to read the words when they appear in stories; the teacher must explicitly have students read these words in text if he or she wants students to generalize the new recognition to connected text. Therefore, whether the teacher is aligning instruction to facilitate skill acquisition or fluency, he or she should always emphasize generalization by teaching students to use newly acquired reading skills across words with lots of examples, different texts, across time, and in comprehension activities. Strategies that teachers can use to promote proficiency at each level of the learning hierarchy are listed in Table 2.2. When you are evaluating a child in a classroom context, ask yourself whether the student is at the acquisition or the fluency stage. If there are many incorrect responses, he or she is probably just acquiring the skill. If there are many correct answers but each takes a long time or if decoding the words takes a long time, then you know that the student needs to work on fluency. This model represents one way to determine whether student proficiency and teaching methods are appropriately aligned. Instructional procedures that are misaligned with the student's level of proficiency (e.g., independent practice is assigned when the student is not accurate) will not improve, and will probably hinder, student learning.

Prerequisite Skills

If the student is at the acquisition stage, an even more basic question that you should be asking is whether the student has the prerequisite skills necessary to learn the newly targeted skill (Howell & Nolet, 2000; Wolery, Bailey, & Sugai, 1988). Indeed, a student's prior knowledge is the best predictor of how much he or she will learn during a lesson (Howell & Nolet, 2000). If prerequisite skills have not been learned, the teacher will either need to teach an easier version of the skill (e.g., teaching just short-*a* vowels rather than teaching all the short vowels together) or an easier skill altogether (e.g., teaching segmenting and blending skills before phonics; Wolery et al., 1988).

Teaching Materials and Difficulty Levels

Examining the instructional materials used to teach students will help you considerably in determining the appropriateness of instruction. We recommend that when you first walk into a classroom (or even before), you carefully examine the materials and instructional

TABLE 2.2. The Instructional Hierarchy: Aligning Instructional Practices with Student Levels of Proficiency

Proficiency level	Characteristic performance	Instructional strategies
Acquisition	Student working on accurate answers	Demonstration/modeling; prompting correct answers; error correction; feedback for every response
Fluency	Student answers are accurate but slow	Practice; incentives for speed; feedback after multiple student responses (e.g., whole worksheet completed)
Generalization	Student working on accurate and fluent performance	Practice and feedback across instructional items (e.g., reading many long-vowel words); practicing the skill across similar types of instructional items (e.g., reading long-*a* and long-*e* words); explicitly teaching the student when, and when not, to use the skill and assigning practice (e.g., reading long-*a* words and short-*a* words); using the skill to perform other skills successfully (e.g., reading long-vowel words in phrases and paragraphs)

activities being used for teaching reading. Asking yourself the right questions will help you to "get a handle" on how well the classroom is meeting students' needs. Table 2.3 outlines where you should direct your attention and the key questions you should ask. The difficulty level of instructional tasks reflects whether the student is appropriately placed in the curriculum. Is the student mostly accurate in his or her responses? If not, he or she should be. Gickling and Rosenfield (1995) recommend that students' accuracy during reading instruction should be between 93 and 97%. They also recommend that accuracy should be 70–85% for practice exercises. When student accuracy is not up to these levels during reading instruction (including reading aloud and guided practice), task difficulty level is probably too high; tasks need to be regulated so that students can achieve more success (Gickling & Rosenfield, 1995). When task difficulty level is appropriate, other problems are forestalled. For example, when the student is able to do most of the work accurately, he or she does not have the time to misbehave in the classroom. For these reasons, we recom-

TABLE 2.3. What You Need to Do and What You Need to Ask to Understand the Impact of the Classroom on Student Learning

Your "to-do" list . . .	Inquire through asking and observing . . .
• Find out whether the child is at the acquisition or fluency stage with the skill(s) on which he or she is currently working.	Are there frequent incorrect answers? Are answers correct but slow?
• Examine the instructional activities and determine whether there is a match or mismatch between student proficiency level and instructional methods.	Does instruction target the appropriate types of student responses (e.g., segmenting and blending sounds, letter–sound correspondences, reading fluency, comprehension)? Are the instructional procedures (e.g., modeling, practice) appropriate for this level of proficiency? Is the difficulty level appropriate? Are enough examples and instructional items presented and is there a variety of examples and nonexamples? Does the student actually have to use the skill to get the right answer? Is the range and sequence of responses sufficient to guarantee that the student will be able to perform the skill in the future and with similar examples he or she hasn't yet encountered?
• Consider how instruction is sequenced.	Is modeling of new skills followed by guided practice, and then by independent practice? Is there a criterion of some sort (other than the passage of time) for deciding when the student has learned the new skill and that it is time to move to the next target? Is the teacher actively promoting the generalization of newly acquired skills to other texts, across time, and to improve comprehension?
• Check to see how skills are being monitored.	Is there adequate feedback or assessment information that tells the teacher what to do next, based on how the student is currently doing?

mend that you consider which skill is being targeted for instruction and whether or not the activities are at an appropriate instructional level for students.

Other Qualities of Teaching Materials

When examining the instructional materials and activities, it is not sufficient to note whether the students are working on alphabetics, phonics, fluency, or comprehension tasks with a high degree of accuracy. The quality of the instructional activities also impacts student performance, and the selection and sequencing of examples and instructional items affects the rate of learning (Kinder & Carnine, 1991). While teaching a new skill, the instructional materials used should present a wide variety of examples and applications that differ from each other as much as possible, while still exemplifying the skill being taught. For example, when teaching students how to read words with *a* as the short vowel, many different words with short *a* should be presented (e.g., *mad, bat, fan*). This variety helps students apply the skill of reading short *a* to future words (i.e., generalization). Students must learn to not overuse particular skills, however. To help students avoid this problem, instructional materials should include nonexamples that *resemble* bona fide examples but differ in the critical attribute that makes them different. For instance, when teaching how to read long-*a* words like *fade*, nonexamples like *fad* should be interspersed during the lesson. As a nonexample, *fad* resembles *fade* in every way except for the critical attribute that distinguishes them (i.e., *e* following the consonant *d*). This step helps students to learn when to use the skill and when not to use the skill.

The final point to look for when you are examining the instructional materials and activities is whether students actually get to practice the skill that is being taught. Although this sounds obvious, it is not; there are many curricular materials that provide additional "hints" or that allow students to get the right answer for the wrong reason (Vargas, 1984). This principle hit home for one of us (EJD) when, while looking over the shoulder of one of his daughters who was doing a homework exercise on writing numbers in 1's and 10's columns, he became aware, through questioning, that she had figured out where to put the numbers without even being able to read the double-digit numbers! Though this example is not directly related to reading, you need not look far for direct examples. When students can fill in the blanks for vocabulary words embedded in definitions based on the number of letters in the word, they are certainly not learning vocabulary words.

The most common source of reading materials is basal reading packages. Basal readers contain texts and instructional activities that guide teachers in reading instruction by providing "instructional manuals . . . with detailed lesson plans and activities for the whole school year, and accompanying reading and lesson materials for students" (National Research Council, 1998, p. 189). The NRC report demonstrates that because (1) new editions are revised based on market research, (2) revisions occur every 3 to 5 years, and (3) there is a time lag between preferred instructional practices and when they appear in new reading series. Analyses of the content of basal reading packages indicate that there is wide variability in their recommendations for such instructional activities as reading aloud to kindergartners, blending and segmenting activities, teaching sound–symbol relationships, use of text that is decodable according to conventions of phonics, and even writing (Adams, 1990; National Research Council, 1998). Another problem with basal reading packages is that to handle the diversity of reading skills in classrooms, most basal reading series either present a wide selection of optional activities or give directions to have students choose activities (National Research Council, 1998). As a result, the teacher receives little explicit guidance in how to teach effectively so that all students can learn. The report's sobering analysis of basal readers is nothing short of scathing:

> Programs that ignore necessary instructional components tacitly delegate the pedagogical support on which their sales are predicated to the intervention of teachers, tutors, or parents. Even when a program does address key instructional components, it may or may not do so with clarity or effect. In this vein, a particular problem is the currently popular publishing strategy of accommodating the range of student interests and teacher predilections by providing activities to please everyone in each lesson. By making it impossible for teachers to pursue all suggestions, the basal programs make it necessary for teachers to ignore some of them. A good basal program should clearly distinguish key from optional activities. (p. 207)

It's obviously not safe to assume that the reading curriculum being used will guide the teacher in knowing how to respond to the referred student's reading problem.

Summarizing with an Example

To summarize the dimensions of effective instruction discussed thus far and to highlight a few others that are also important to the delivery of instruction, we will put all these principles in the context of Mrs. Walker's reading class. Mrs. Walker could be teaching virtually any of the elementary grades. She should be doing the following things, regardless of the grade level. First, Mrs. Walker chooses appropriate tasks and adjusts the difficulty to obtain the optimal ratio of correct answers to incorrect answers. If skills that are prerequisites to what she intends to teach have not been learned, she modifies her lesson plan to teach the prerequisites. When she introduces activities, she explains why the students are working on them, thereby maintaining a cognitive focus in her classroom (Ysseldyke & Christenson, 1993). Additionally, she gives clear instructions for how to complete the task along with a description of incentives for finishing work accurately (e.g., "When you are done with your seatwork assignment, you may have time in the play area").

When she is teaching a new skill, she shows students how to do the skill (providing modeling), and offers opportunities for guided practice with immediate feedback for performance. Mrs. Walker maintains a brisk pace when instructing by presenting instructional material rapidly enough so students don't have time to fool around and are accountable to give answers frequently (Carnine, 1976). Mrs. Walker directly teaches students to discriminate when to use the newly learned skill and when to not use the newly learned skill. To achieve the latter, she carefully sequences items so that there is both variety and nonexamples. In addition, she gives rules for when to use the skill, if appropriate. During guided practice Mrs. Walker has students articulate the rules to be sure they are learning them. Once students have achieved accuracy in the use of the skill, she provides ample practice with feedback about performance to promote fluency. To help students generalize the newly learned skill, Mrs. Walker has them use the skill with many different types of problems and in the context of other skills and "real world" applications. Under these conditions we expect to see high levels of *active student engagement*, including writing, reading aloud, silent reading, asking and answering academic questions, academic game play, and discussion about the subject matter (Greenwood, Terry, Marquis, & Walker, 1994). Finally, Mrs. Walker moves on in the curriculum only when she sees evidence that the students have actually learned the skill and can use it in meaningful ways.

Of course, Mrs. Walker has a diversity of skills-related needs in her classroom, so she has a lot to manage at one time. Like many teachers, Mrs. Walker uses instructional groupings to meet this diversity of needs. However, decisions about issues such as whether to move students on in the curriculum depend on how well each individual student responds to her teaching (and not just the passage of time). She demonstrates sensitivity to students' needs by altering instruction based on how well they handle the demands placed on them.

Sufficient Time for Learning and Meaningful Active Engagement

Teachers must devote sufficient time to reading instruction (Gettinger, 1995). Better teachers devote more time to instruction (Rosenshine, 1980). Because time is not sufficient in itself, however, students must also be actively engaged in reading (Gettinger, 1995). If 2 hours are scheduled for language arts but the referred student spends only 4 minutes reading during the 2-hour period, then the student is not likely to become a good reader any time soon. You will note that instructional procedures and materials discussed up to this point either prompt the student to respond in some way or provide feedback to the student regarding his or her responses. Classrooms where students are busy but little reading is going on are not making the most of the time available for reading instruction.

Responsive Instruction

Obviously, instruction involves more than just presenting activities from a curriculum or basal reading series in sequence. Yet, it can turn into this kind of rote activity if decisions are based on the passage of time (e.g., the teacher teaches one story per week regardless of how students do with the story) or pressures to move through the curriculum at a certain pace in order to finish before the end of the school year. Problems can occur for other reasons as well. Instruction must be based on what students already know, how proficient they are with current objectives, and how well they are progressing in response to the teacher's efforts. Otherwise, students won't learn. Effective instruction is *responsive* to students, beginning with the skills or lack of skills they bring to the classroom and the progress they are making or not making after instruction has begun. For instruction to be responsive, there must be a feedback loop whereby the teacher gets solid and reliable feedback about whether the student has truly learned what was taught. The student's behavior should signal to the teacher what to do next (Daly & Murdoch, 2000). When there is a lack of good information about what the student knows, has learned, and is learning, a better monitoring system or feedback loop is needed, and instruction should be realigned with the student's needs. Therefore, checking out how the teacher monitors students is a necessary step. If there is no systematic monitoring going on, putting a system in place is an important first step.

As you take this approach, you may hear objections that teachers don't and can't provide instruction for an individual student. True. However, teachers *do* and *must* (1) make instructional decisions for each and every student in the classroom, and (2) deliver instruction to every child in the classroom. The decision to put five children in a small reading group for instruction represents individual decisions for each one of those children (i.e., five decisions). We are certainly not advocating individual instruction for all children. We are, however, advocating instruction that is *responsive to every student's needs*. Otherwise, it's not instruction; it's just presenting curriculum materials. Some students will probably still learn with a standard approach to delivering the curriculum. The student(s) you are worried about, on the other hand, probably won't! The goal is to make the right instructional decisions for *every* child in the classroom. The diversity of student skills that is typical of classrooms requires teachers to do different things for different students, regardless of whether or not they group them for some activities.

IDENTIFYING THE ENTRY POINT
FOR INTERVENTION EFFORTS

All this knowledge about effective instruction and how to facilitate effective interventions for reading problems is useless if the organizational systems of the classroom, the school, and the school district do not have the capacity for change. If some teachers or schools have been unwilling to change to meet the instructional needs of students, President Bush's No Child Left Behind legislation and its effects on states and local school districts may provide just the right motivating conditions necessary to make them more willing to change. No Child Left Behind emphasizes school accountability and empirically proven practices and promises to apply consequences when students don't improve. That said, it would be naïve to assume that this piece of federal legislation alone is sufficient to get unmotivated schools "in gear" and working on the problem. You will not be an effective consultant if you are unable to assess the ability of the organization to change and modify its procedures and adjust your services accordingly. In a broader sense, your consulting responsibilities bring you into contact with at least one organizational system (e.g., a school), which, like an individual human being, has its own needs and limitations (Skrtic, 1991). It would be unwise to forge ahead with an intervention and ignore the organizational structure, needs, and limitations of the school system. The most salient factors that will affect (positively or adversely) the likelihood of developing a successful intervention include (1) the frequency of reading problems in the classroom, school, and school district, (2) available resources for intervention, and (3) whether intervention is truly an organizational priority for the classroom, school, and district. We have identified potential stumbling blocks that may affect a school's capacity for change; Table 2.4 lists reasons why con-

**TABLE 2.4. Stumbling Blocks
to Effective Consultation**

1. Too much effort for too little yield
2. Unsound instructional environment
3. Conflicting organizational priorities
4. Unwillingness to cooperate
5. The right questions are not being asked

sultants may be ineffective in their attempts to help schools intervene with reading problems.

Too Much Effort for Too Little Yield

In many cases, designing individualized interventions for each and every child who is having a reading problem may be an overwhelming task. The first question that you must ask yourself is whether the referred child is one of only a few cases or whether this child is representative of the problems of many children in the system (i.e., classroom, school, or school district). In other words, is this a low-rate problem or a high-rate problem? If it is a high-rate problem, individualized assessments and interventions will be costly and time consuming—and not the most effective approach. In this case, a more efficient and defensible approach is to adopt a validated reading program and apply it to the school or the district. Proven strategies such as Direct Instruction and Success for All, which are instructional methods that replace typical basal reading approaches, are likely to improve the instruction that the students are receiving and reduce the need for expensive diagnostic procedures that must be administered to students who are failing, or at risk for failing, thereby making it more cost effective overall (Adelman, 1982). You can obtain more information about Direct Instruction by visiting the website of the National Institute for Direct Instruction at *http://www.nifti.org/*. Information about Success for All can be found at *http://successforall.com/*. The school or district is likely to produce better effects by investing in a program that has been proven to be effective and reserving time and resource-consuming diagnostic practices for the children who do not improve when the newly adopted instructional program is in place. This is precisely what No Child Left Behind prescribes.

If the incidence of reading problems in the school is not widespread, then we suggest the individual kind of analysis described throughout the rest of the book. A more careful examination of the individual circumstances of the reading problem will reveal the mismatch between the child's instructional needs and how classroom instruction is arranged and delivered. Fortunately, the assessment methods described in the latter chapters are simple and time efficient, making them appropriate for group administration in most circumstances. The assessor can evaluate all the children in a classroom or a representative sample in a school building in far less time than it takes to conduct an eligibility determination assessment for a single child. By looking for all students who could benefit from intervention, you can quickly gauge whether an individualized or a group intervention is warranted.

Unsound Instructional Environment

In a poorly managed classroom, newly devised intervention procedures will quickly become a burden to the teacher. Unfortunately, many teachers are ill prepared to teach reading. As noted in Chapter 1, the average number of courses on reading instruction taken by teachers is only 1.3 (National Reading Council, 1998). Effective reading instruction involves more than simply following the activities outlined in a basal reader. Although inservice teacher education can generally improve student achievement (National Reading Panel, 2000), the fact that so little money is allocated by districts for this purpose, combined with the variable quality of the teacher inservice education that is provided (National Reading Council, 1998), reduces the chances of the inservice model truly improving teacher performance. Our intention is not to disparage teachers' abilities but to give a realistic perspective on how ill prepared some teachers might be to teach reading effectively.

When classroom instruction is not well managed, you are faced with a dilemma. Pursuing a child-focused, individualized reading intervention may help the child and "fill in the gaps" where current reading instruction is not doing the job. However, if the teacher has difficulty managing instruction in the first place, will he or she be able to manage an additional intervention on top of what is being done ineffectively? If, on the other hand, you work with the teacher to facilitate a more general intervention to improve the overall planning and delivery of reading instruction, improvements in the class structure and delivery of instruction for the whole class may or may not pay off for the individually referred child. In other words, if you can get the teacher to use higher quality materials, improve the clarity of directions and instruction, and improve guided practice and feedback for the class as a whole, this may still not be enough for the individual child about whom you are consulting.

Given that there are advantages and disadvantages to both tactics, we feel that the best approach in this situation is to help the teacher improve the overall instruction in the classroom. If the teacher is able to change instruction but the target child does not improve, the fact that the teacher successfully implemented a new instructional program should increase your confidence that he or she can make other changes successfully as well. You should then work to develop a more individualized intervention to meet that child's needs. Furthermore, other children will benefit from the improved instruction.

Conflicting Organizational Priorities

Schools' priorities may actually hamper intervention efforts. This problem can manifest itself in several forms. District-adopted curricular materials may not be the most effective materials for teaching reading. Districts may be wooed into adopting a new or revised reading program that reflects the most popular educational trend but doesn't provide sufficient guidance in effective instruction to teachers. Very few basal reading programs actually structure lessons carefully enough to allow students to truly master the material (Adams, 1990; National Reading Council, 1998).

Desire to change is not enough. Tangible support must be put behind that desire. Schools might recognize a need for intervention, but administrative support may be weak. If, for example, administrators are not willing to provide teachers with support so that they have time to consult and problem solve or receive adequate training, teachers won't become more effective. Tangible support must also be directed in the right way. Education tends to be fad oriented. Giving teachers release time so that they can go to inservice training on the latest reading instruction method won't help anyone if that method is not backed by good scientific research. Schools need to increase their standards for what constitutes an effective intervention. Indeed, No Child Left Behind mandates it.

Unwillingness to Cooperate

Schools or teachers may be unwilling to cooperate with efforts to design effective reading interventions. In that case, you will spare all involved a lot of tension and headaches if you help the school or teacher understand that *your* ability to help is severely limited when there is a lack of a shared desire to make the plan work. It is necessary to understand that there may be other rewards accruing to teachers who refuse to cooperate. For instance, if referral for evaluation has generally led to students being identified as learning disabled and removed (at least partially) from the classroom, then you are asking the teacher to do more work by engaging in a consultation process that will involve classroom modifications, when the alternative (i.e., removal from the classroom) involves less work and responsibility. Even very effective teachers will probably feel some relief when a student is identified as learning disabled, because the label at least partially absolves the teacher from responsibility, and it means that someone else will be taking charge of the child's instruction.

The Right Questions Are Not Being Asked

The problem of not asking the right questions is related to the prior problem of uncooperativeness. Unfortunately, schools have set up a categorical system for identifying problems that describes them as occurring *within* the child. School psychologists and other educators spend a significant amount of time trying to diagnose what's wrong with *the child*. The focus is on asking, "How do we diagnose whether the child has a problem and what kind of problem is it?" A more productive approach is to ask (1) why there is a problem in this particular classroom, (2) what we can do about it (based on the results), and (3) how we can show whether modifications improved reading performance or not. An effective consultant frames the critical questions in terms of the interaction between a learner and his or her environment and then gathers information to identify the locus of the mismatch. When designing an intervention, the effective consultant should be asking:

Who will be doing the intervention?
How do we know that this person is adequately trained?

How do we know that the person is, in fact, doing the intervention correctly? How do we show whether it is effective or not?

The remainder of this book deals with how to frame the problem-solving process within these question frameworks and, more importantly, how to go about answering them.

INTERNET RESOURCES

We have identified a number of resources on the Internet that can support your intervention efforts and supplement the model (with materials and intervention ideas) that is presented in this book. The following websites give information about effective instruction, identifying effective reading interventions, or gathering materials for monitoring student outcomes.

Dynamic Indicators of Basic Early Literacy Skills (DIBELS)

DIBELS is a set of methods and materials for assessing early literacy, fluency, and comprehension skills. Developed by researchers at the University of Oregon, DIBELS has become popular nationally with school districts that are trying to live up to the requirements of the No Child Left Behind Act. The website contains free assessment materials as well as assessment and scoring rules that can be downloaded. Printed copies of materials are available for a fee. A large national database is available to users who wish to compare their students' performance to other students' scores. Through the DIBELS data system, quarterly reports for students, classes, schools, and districts can be generated for a small fee ($1 per student per year, at the time of this writing). The website even has video clips demonstrating proper administration methods. There are many links to other useful literacy sites. The website address is *http://dibels.uoregon.edu*.

Edformation

Edformation is described as a "fluency company." It offers products and services related to reading fluency assessments (discussed in Chapters 2 and 3), the results of which can be evaluated online. The online service even prompts instructional decisions when sufficient data have been gathered. These materials and services, available for a fee, will allow you to do many of the things that are discussed in the following chapters. The Edformation website address is *http://www.edformation.com/*.

Headsprout

Headsprout is a reading instruction program in which students are taught to read in 40 lessons on the Internet. It is heavily based on explicit teaching of phonics. The designers of this program have been using fluency-based instruction very effectively for a number of years (especially for students with high-incidence disabilities, such as learning disabilities and attention-deficit/hyperactivity disorder). Check it out at *http://headsprout.com*.

Institute for the Development of Educational Achievement (IDEA)

IDEA is an initiative by researchers at the University of Oregon whose purpose is to increase awareness of empirically valid reading interventions and to build schools' capacity for incorporating effective assessment and reading intervention programs. You will find information about and links to intervention programs (e.g., the Optimize Intervention program for improving phonemic segmenting and blending skills) that can be adopted on a classroom or schoolwide basis, evaluations of assessment instruments, presentations on implementation of effective reading programs (with very specific examples of how to interpret assessment results through the link to the Institute on Beginning Reading), and DIBELS (described earlier). You can find it at *http://idea.uoregon.edu/*.

Intervention Central

This website contains many resources for creating a wide variety of curriculum-based measurement materials (including a manual for how to use curriculum-based measurement and various readability formulas for determining the difficulty level of reading passages), intervention strategies, and information for improving the functioning of school-based intervention teams. Curriculum-based measurement is a popular and valid fluency assessment method that is covered in detail in the following chapters. You can find it at *http://www.interventioncentral.org*.

National Reading Panel

The NRP report gives a comprehensive overview of empirical reading research across the full spectrum of reading skills. You can use the information to identify empirically validated intervention strategies. You can find the report at *http://www.nichd.nih.gov/publications/nrp/smallbook.htm*.

3

Selecting and Monitoring
Early Literacy Interventions

Early literacy skills are the building blocks of reading success. A substantial literature base has emphasized the importance of establishing early literacy skills in order to become a successful, fluent reader (see Adams, 1990). Clear documentation has emerged that a lack of these skills distinguishes poor from good readers. Failure to obtain early literacy skills creates a domino effect that decreases the likelihood of achieving grade-level reading skill. In addition, deficits in early literacy skills persist, meaning that they can be found in older children and adults who are poor readers (Pratt & Brady, 1988). As a result of increased knowledge about the importance of early literacy skill acquisition, information and related materials regarding these skills have proliferated in the literature. This chapter brings together that information to provide a concise understanding of how to effectively assess and intervene at the initial stages of reading acquisition.

Early literacy skills lead the young child to develop understanding of the *alphabetic principle*, which is one crucial step to becoming a successful reader. The alphabetic principle refers to the notion that one symbol (i.e., a letter) corresponds to each basic speech sound in language. Once this connection has been learned, it is possible for the learner to combine symbols and sounds to read the words that are commonly spoken. As was pointed out in Chapter 2, it is this connection that allows a student to then work on becoming an accurate and fluent reader. However, the simplicity of the concept is somewhat deceiving. The alphabetic principle can be complicated and difficult for many learners to grasp, because the significance of a letter is often modified by its surrounding letters. That is, each letter does not correspond neatly with only one sound, but can change in the context of various combinations. For example, the letter *c* makes a different sound in *cat, city,* and *chat*. Thus, it is not easy for many beginning readers to comprehend the alphabetic principle. Establishing this understanding is dependent on many early literacy skills, with fluent letter naming and awareness of phonemes being two of the most important skills (Adams, 1990). Discussion of each of these skills and their relation to reading frames the major portion of this chapter.

WHAT IS EARLY LITERACY?

Definition

One of the first tasks to understanding the selection and monitoring of early literacy interventions is to define the term. *Early literacy* typically refers to discrete "basic" skills that are foundational to fluent reading. Researchers have examined skills such as letter knowledge, phonological awareness, concepts of print, and naming of letters, colors, and objects to determine acquisition rates and prediction of later achievement (e.g., Blachman, 1994; Daly, Wright, Kelly, & Martens, 1997; Walsh, Price, & Gillingham, 1988). This body of work most frequently references two skills as strong predictors of reading achievement: phonological awareness and letter knowledge. Early literacy, however, should not be confused with *emergent literacy*, which refers to a broader concept of literacy that begins before formal instruction and leads to awareness and knowledge of print (Gunn, Simmons, & Kame'enui, 1995). Specific areas contained within the more inclusive concept of emergent literacy are identified in Table 3.1. Although important in their own right, limited experimental research is available regarding the areas that comprise emergent literacy.

TABLE 3.1. **Areas of Emergent Literacy**

Area	Definition	Examples
Awareness of print	Knowledge of the conventions, purposes, and uses of print	Print, not pictures, tells the story or provides a message. Writing creates a story.
Relationship of print to speech	Understanding the physical, situational, and structural differences between oral and written language	Oral conversation is distinguished from a "read" news item. Oral language expresses and explores, whereas written language prompts comparison and analysis. Speech is more informal than writing.
Comprehension of text structures	Knowledge about grammar and organization of stories	Opening and closing phrases, such as "once upon a time," are recognized.
Phonological awareness	Sensitivity to the sounds in oral language	Early skills include rhyming, alliteration, and sentence segmentation.
Letter knowledge	Knowledge of the alphabet and related sounds	The child is exposed to and "plays games" with alphabet books, blocks, and shapes.

Note. Data from Gunn et al. (1995).

This chapter focuses on the more discrete skills described as early literacy. A brief description of each skill covered in this chapter appears in Table 3.2. These are the skills children are expected to master during the first few years of formal schooling. Providing explicit instruction in phonological awareness and letter knowledge has produced impressive results across multiple dimensions (e.g., grades, ages, classrooms; National Reading Panel, 2000). These skills can be defined in observable and measurable terms, are responsive to instruction, and, as noted earlier, serve as the foundation for later reading skills, making them common targets for assessment and instruction. A review of our current understanding of these critical early literacy skills—phonological awareness and letter knowledge—is presented next.

Phonological Awareness

What Is It?

Phonological awareness refers to a sensitivity to the sounds or phonological segments in a spoken word as well as the ability to manipulate those segments. It is important to remember that phonological awareness is a form of sensitivity to oral language that manifests itself in the absence of written language. It encompasses a broad range of skills that can be hierarchically arranged by difficulty. For example, beginning phonological awareness may include skill with rhyming or identifying similar word beginnings or endings. Later phonological awareness requires greater, or more explicit, manipulation of sounds. This is when the term *phonemic*, rather than phonological awareness, is applicable, because attention is explicitly focused on understanding and direct manipulation of individual sounds. For example, segmenting (breaking a word into each sound), blending (putting sounds together to form a word), and deleting sounds are skills requiring a higher level of phonological awareness. An example of skill progression in phonological awareness is presented in Table 3.3.

Phonological awareness is only one of the skills within a framework of *phonological processing* abilities. Phonological processing includes at least three kinds of skills: phonological awareness, phonological coding, and retrieval of phonological codes (Torgesen,

TABLE 3.2. Review of Key Terms

Early literacy	Discrete "basic" skills that are built upon as the child becomes a fluent reader
Phonological awareness	Sensitivity to the sounds or phonological segments in a spoken word as well as the ability to manipulate those segments
Phonological processing	Includes the three abilities of phonological awareness, phonological codes, and retrieval of phonological codes
Alphabetic principle	Each symbol (letter) corresponds to each basic sound in speech; also referred to as letter–sound correspondences
Letter-naming fluency	Accurate and rapid naming of letters

TABLE 3.3. **Hierarchy of Phonological Awareness Skills: Possible Activities and Examples**

Rhyme	Providing	"Tell me another word that rhymes with *bat*."
	Categorizing	"Which word does not rhyme with *bat—cat, big,* or *sat*?"
	Judging	"Do *bat* and *cat* rhyme?"
Alliteration	Providing	"What is the first sound in *bat*?"
	Categorizing	"Which word has the same first sound as *bat—big, sat,* or *pet*?"
	Judging	"Do *bat* and *big* have the same first sound?"
Blending	One or two sounds	"What word does /p/-/at/ make?"
	Entire word	"What word does /p/-/a/-/t/ make?"
Segmentation	Count	"How many sounds do you hear in the word *sit*?"
	Tap	"Tap your finger for each sound in the word *sit*."
	Name	"Tell me the sounds you hear in *sit*."
Manipulation	Deletion	"If you take away the /s/ in *sit*, what is left?"
	Substitution	"Change the /n/ sound in *net* to /b/. What is the new word?"
	Reversal	"Reverse the sounds in *net*. What is the new word?"

Wagner, & Rashotte, 1994). *Phonological coding* refers to the ability to hold phonological information in working memory; it is often assessed with memory span tasks (i.e., repeating nonmeaningful sequences of verbal items). *Retrieval of phonological codes*, or rate of access to phonological information, is typically measured by rapid naming tasks (letters, digits, colors, objects). It has been suggested that all of the phonological processing skills may be important in explaining differences in responsiveness to intervention, and the degree to which each ability is amenable to change is uncertain. Although some phonological processing abilities may be fairly stable, we do know that phonological awareness can be taught. As Blachman (1994) pointed out, simply because some students respond more to instructional efforts does not negate the need for intervention; rather, it implies that different levels or types of intervention may be needed for different students.

When Is It Typically Acquired?

Rudimentary phonological awareness skills can be evident in preschool children as young as 2 or 3 years old. For example, studies have found that children as young as 3 years possess some awareness of rhymes (McLean, Bryant, & Bradley, 1987) and sentence or syllable segmentation (Fox & Routh, 1975). More advanced phonological awareness typically becomes evident during the first few years of formal school and is generally well established by second grade. A number of researchers have suggested that the greatest increases in phonological awareness occur between kindergarten and first grade (Chafouleas, Lewandowski, Smith, & Blachman, 1997; Fox & Routh, 1975; Liberman, Shankweiler, Fischer, & Carter, 1974). One study found that most phonological awareness tasks were generally mastered (90% correct) by the age of 7 years (Chafouleas et al., 1997).

Our general understanding of the relationship between phonological awareness and reading is that some beginning phonological awareness is needed to facilitate reading. Once reading begins to be established, a reciprocal relationship is fueled: Each promotes the other. Given that reading success seems to hinge, in part, on having phonological awareness, the early elementary years certainly present a sensitive period for instruction and skill acquisition. In fact, although phonological awareness can be developed in students after this period, "reading" time lost during that period is difficult to compensate for. Older students have to work harder to catch up, and missed reading time during those early years may make reading a more laborious task in the long run for them.

Letter Knowledge

What Is It?

In contrast to the oral nature of phonological awareness, letter knowledge refers to orthographic skill—that is, knowledge of the written symbols that represent the sounds in language. This knowledge can be demonstrated in a variety of ways, from accurate naming of letters to fluent (accurate and rapid) naming of letters. In addition, letter knowledge can refer to learning letter sounds. Although the literature has not determined if it is best to teach letter names, letter sounds, or both (Stahl, Duffy-Hester, & Stahl, 1998), we do know that letter knowledge is an important early literacy skill. Letter-naming fluency, in particular, has been found to be a good indicator or predictor of reading achievement (Daly et al., 1997; Kaminski & Good, 1996). We also know, however, that simply teaching letter naming alone is probably not sufficient to ensure reading success. A combination of letter knowledge and phonological awareness forms the core requirements of understanding the alphabetic principle.

When Is It Typically Acquired?

The acquisition of alphabet knowledge typically involves a gradual accumulation of letter knowledge from 3 to 7 years of age (Worden & Boettcher, 1990). In addition, research has suggested that the speed with which letters are named, not only the naming of them, is important (e.g., Blachman, 1994; Walsh et al., 1988). For example, findings have suggested that rapid naming of letters and words can differentiate good and poor readers, with weaker readers demonstrating slower naming speeds. This finding seems logical in that, when learning most skills, a student first works on performing accurately and then moves to performing both accurately and quickly.

Understanding How It All Goes Together

Although the relationship among various early literacy skills and reading skill is far from being fully understood, the simple consensus is that children must have a basic understanding that words are made of different sounds (i.e., phonological awareness) prior to being able to understand letter–sound correspondences (i.e., the alphabetic principle) necessary to decode unfamiliar words. In other words, students need to possess a minimum amount of phonological awareness before they will be able to use letter-name knowledge (Tunmer, Herriman, & Nesdale, 1988). Thus, a basic rule of instruction is to teach these discrete skills in a properly sequenced fashion (i.e., easiest to hardest), such as single letters with limited possible pronunciations to multiletter sound units or letters with multiple pronunciations (Adams, 1990). Once basic phonological awareness and letter knowledge skills have been acquired, the child has the foundation upon which to understand and apply the alphabetic principle. The child can then devote more energy to understanding the connections, without having to stop to remember which name or sound goes with which symbol. Fluency, or automaticity with phonemic skills and letter recognition, is the ultimate goal of this phase of the process of learning to read.

The discrete skills discussed thus far do not represent a complete reading curriculum. These skills were selected and emphasized because they represent good indicators of early reading and thus should be taught explicitly. However, other skills and other methods of exposing students to the skills should be included. For example, these early literacy skills can be emphasized through methods other than teaching in isolation (e.g., looking at patterns without interference). Students can be exposed through mediums such as meaningful and interesting stories and writing (dictation and invented spelling; Smith, Simmons, & Kame'enui, 1995).

WHY IS PROFICIENCY WITH EARLY LITERACY SKILLS DIFFICULT FOR SOME STUDENTS TO ACHIEVE?

There are two primary reasons why students struggle to obtain early literacy skills: (1) lack of adequate exposure to appropriate instruction, and (2) stable individual characteristics that suggest a need for more intensive early literacy instruction.

First, students may have difficulty obtaining early literacy skills because they have either not had enough instruction or the appropriate types of instruction. Early literacy skills, particularly phonological awareness, can be difficult to achieve without explicit, systematic instruction. Even for a normally achieving child, it is challenging to think of words as individual sounds. The phoneme is an abstract unit of speech. In addition, phonemes are co-articulated—that is, they sound like one unit—making it even more difficult to differentiate discrete sounds. In fact, there are 44 different phonemes within the English language. The lack of a one-to-one correspondence between the letters that appear on a page and the sounds they make when articulated as phonemes creates ambiguities for the learner. For example, *shirt*, a five-letter word, has only four phonemes because the /sh/ is one phoneme (i.e., sound). Similarly, *cow*, a three-letter word, has only two phonemes due to the /ow/ combination. Furthermore, difficulty in understanding phonemes can vary by the type and number of sounds (Chafouleas, VanAuken, & Dunham, 2001; McBride-Chang, 1995) and even the type of task, as discussed earlier. For example, it has generally been found that sounds that can be held (i.e., *continuant* sounds, such as /s/) are easier to grasp than sounds that cannot (i.e., *stop* sounds, such as /t/). In addition, the fewer the sounds, the better. That is, generally two- or three-phoneme words are easier to grasp than four-phoneme words, and memory difficulties can arise with words containing more than four phonemes (McBride-Chang, 1995).

The second explanation for difficulty in obtaining early literacy skills comes from research suggesting there may be stable individual characteristics that warrant differential instruction. As discussed earlier, phonological awareness is only one of the skills encompassed under phonological processing. The other skills—phonological coding and retrieval of phonological codes—are both related to memory and appear to be relatively stable or at least resistant to change. This line of research suggests that even with a curriculum that includes explicit instruction in phonological awareness and letter knowledge, all students may not acquire early literacy skills at the same rate. This differential learning means that instruction in phonological awareness and letter knowledge may need to be modified or intensified for some students.

HOW SHOULD WE ASSESS EARLY LITERACY?

Characteristics of a Good Assessment Technique

Although not specifically addressing the assessment of early literacy, Fuchs and Fuchs (1999) offered relevant criteria for evaluating measures of reading. First, reliability (consistency), validity, and accuracy of the assessment tools should be examined. For example, degree of reliability can vary in relation to the range of test scores, difficulty of test items, and the probability of guessing the correct answer. In one investigation, measures requiring a student to *produce* a response were found to have better characteristics than those requiring *selection* of a response (Daly et al., 1997). For example, take a rhyming task using the word *sand*. The task could be structured to have the student produce another word that rhymes with *sand* (production response), or the student could be asked to select from four pictures the one picture that does (or does not) rhyme with *sand* (selection response).

Second, the tools should be sensitive to instructional effects over time and empower educators to make changes in instruction when the student is not learning. One prerequisite to sensitivity is that the task should be hard enough to reveal areas in which performance could improve, but not so hard that few items can be answered. If no items can be answered correctly, it will probably be difficult to determine the specific type of instruction that is needed. For example, as discussed in the section on acquiring phonological awareness, providing or identifying the first sound in a word is typically an easier task than segmenting an entire word. Thus, if a student can already segment initial sounds, assessment of that skill would not be meaningful. Conversely, if a student does not demonstrate any understanding of segmentation, then an easier task may be more appropriate. In addition, it is important to keep in mind that early literacy skills are generally established quickly and early in a student's school career. Once a student demonstrates progress on early literacy tasks, it may be appropriate to assess reading skills such as oral reading fluency additionally or concurrently (Kaminski & Good, 1996). This issue is addressed further in the next section.

Finally, and perhaps most importantly for the school-based practitioner, the tools must be feasible. They should be efficient to administer and easy to score. Additionally, management of the data for potentially large numbers of students should not be overly cumbersome (Kaminiski & Good, 1996). These considerations offer a useful framework for evaluating various early literacy assessment tools. Worksheet 3.1 (all worksheets are at the end of the chapter) is a useful evaluation tool.

Selecting an Assessment Technique

Given increased knowledge and interest in the area of early literacy, a number of assessment measures has been popping up, leaving questions regarding the appropriate selection of a technique. In addition to the above characteristics, selection of a specific assessment technique depends on the purpose of the assessment. Two assessment purposes related to intervention are screening and progress monitoring. Although a measure would ideally serve both purposes, many available measures do not. Furthermore, some measures include assessment of a wide range of phonological awareness skills, whereas others may focus on particular skills, which may be too easy or too hard for some students.

One well-known test of phonological awareness is the Rosner Test of Auditory Analysis (Rosner, 1975). This test examines the segmentation of words, syllables, and phonemes as well as phoneme deletion. Students are asked to provide production-type responses. Although normative information is not available, information is provided regarding expected performance based on age. Only one form of the measure is available. So, although it may serve as a useful screening tool for a range of segmentation-related skills, its use for repeated assessment over time is limited and specific to the segmentation skill. In contrast, the Comprehensive Test of Phonological Processes (CTOPP; Wagner, Torgesen, & Rashotte, 1999) assesses three broad areas of phonological processing skills (phonological awareness, rapid automatic naming, verbal short-term memory), and norms are available from ages 5 through adulthood. Items within each area are arranged to include both very easy tasks (e.g., syllable segmentation) and harder tasks (e.g., single phoneme deletion), all of which require production-type responses. However, again, although this test has been researched more extensively, only one form is available. Thus, its use for monitoring student performance over time is limited. In addition, administration of the full battery (approximately 20 minutes per student) may not be feasible for large numbers of students. One available test that can be group-administered is the Test of Phonological Awareness (TOPA; Torgesen & Bryant, 1994a). This test can be administered to children in the primary grades (focus is on easy items); it assesses a child's ability to compare first or last sounds when examining four pictures. Thus, the test is limited in that it requires selection-type responses, and again, only one form is available.

As can be noted from these examples, the majority of those measures is primarily useful for screening or pre/post purposes, because only a single form of the measures is available. Thus, the measures do not allow the practitioner to monitor progress incrementally. In addition, administration of the full battery of many measures is often not time efficient. One early literacy assessment system that is an exception to these limitations is the Dynamic Indicators of Early Literacy Skills (DIBELS; Good & Kaminski, 2001). As noted in Chapter 1, DIBELS is a comprehensive, standardized assessment framework for evaluating students' early literacy skills in a variety of areas (phoneme segmentation, initial sounds, letter naming, blending sounds, oral reading fluency). The DIBELS system is popular with school districts across the nation for a number of reasons. First, the measures cover the most critical areas of early literacy skills and provide continuity in assessment. Second, the measures are easy and brief to administer, which makes it possible for a wide variety of individuals (classroom teachers, school psychologists, teaching aides) to administer them. Third, assessment and materials are widely available on the Internet (*http://dibels.uoregon.edu/index.php*) for free or a minimal cost, and online technical support is excellent. Finally, the DIBELS system has a wide variety of uses, comes with benchmarks and norms for student performance on the various measures, and is easily adaptable to ongoing progress monitoring.

With this brief review and suggestions for evaluating available measures, we now turn to describing what we consider an appropriate framework for building assessment devices for two phonological awareness skills (whole-word segmentation and initial sound segmentation) and letter knowledge. This framework and its specific tasks are recommended for a number of reasons. First, the tasks are brief and can be created in multiple forms; thus, the tasks are feasible for use to monitor student progress in school settings. Second, the tasks can help inform instruction because the data indicate appropriate level and type of instruction. Finally, the framework provides flexibility in the selection of tasks so that items can be chosen at the appropriate difficulty level. A continuum of assessment tasks designed to accommodate the needs of nonreaders through beginning readers is provided. First, however, specific procedures and assessment tasks are presented and discussed.

Letter Naming

Assessment of letter-naming skill focuses on providing information about both the accuracy and fluency with which a student can identify correct letter names. Individually administered probes are used to assess the number of correctly read letters a student can orally identify in 1 minute. Each probe is scored based on accuracy (percent correct out of total read) and fluency (rate of correctly read letters). As discussed earlier, fluency with letter naming is a highly predictive skill. General research norms presented by Kaminski and Good (1996) have suggested that students in kindergarten should be able to identify around 28 correct letters per minute, whereas first-grade students should be able to identify more than 60 per minute. Because fluency may be too advanced a standard for some students, accuracy also is calculated. For example, other research (see Stahl & Murray, 1994) has indicated that students need to correctly identify more than 80% of letters in order to be able to learn to manipulate onsets and rimes in words.

Directions for administration of the letter-naming probes as well as five alternate forms can be found in Worksheets 3.2a–f. Additional forms can be easily created with the following guidelines: using a plain piece of paper, randomly select letters, placing five in a row. Letters may be all capital or lowercase, or a combination, as long as the same strategy is used to create all forms. Forms also can be generated at the Intervention Central website (*www.interventioncentral.org*; see Chapter 1).

Phonological Awareness

As with letter naming, scoring can be based on accuracy, fluency, or both. Two tasks were selected as representing appropriate and predictive measures of phonological awareness: whole-word segmentation and initial sound segmentation. Whole-word segmentation requires segmentation of the entire word, whereas initial sound segmentation entails isolating only the first sound in the word. Initial sound segmentation is generally an easier task; it is administered using the same items as the whole-word segmentation task but with different directions. Directions for administration and scoring procedures for creating each of the tasks, as well as enough words to form at least five alternate forms, can be found in Worksheets 3.3a–c. As noted on Worksheet 3.3c, the probes are created by randomly selecting words from the category corresponding to the number of phonemes, until the entire probe sheet is completed. For example, on Worksheet 3.3a, the first item should contain a word from the three-phoneme category. For initial sound segmentation, it is suggested that items be selected from continuant and noncontinuant sound columns alternately, in order to provide approximately equal representation within the probe. Scoring for initial sound segmentation is either correct/incorrect per word, whereas scoring for whole-word segmentation is by correct total segments (e.g., *cat*—possible score of 3). An example of a completed and scored probe for initial sound segmentation can be found in Figure 3.1.

Oral Reading Fluency

The measurement of oral reading fluency presented here follows procedures presented in the literature on curriculum-based measurement for reading (CBM of oral reading; see Shinn, 1989). That is, narrative and expository passages are selected from curriculum materials, and students are asked to read each passage orally for 1 minute. The number of correctly read words per minute is calculated. A correctly read word is defined as a word pronounced correctly within 3 seconds, whereas an error is defined as a word not pronounced correctly within 3 seconds. Omissions, mispronunciations, and hesitations of more than 3 seconds are scored as errors. If the student hesitates for more than 3 seconds, the examiner provides the word and marks it as incorrectly read. Specific procedures and directions can be found in Chapter 4 of this text.

Interpreting the Information

Figure 3.2 presents a flowchart to help guide the selection of appropriate assessment measures and the direction of instructional focus. It is important to note that the numbers in the flowchart present general guidelines for performance only. The numbers represent the level of skill generally to be expected by the end of first grade, unless otherwise noted. Thus, this information also may be used as a reference point when assessing students of other ages and grades. As noted in the flowchart, the first step in assessment is to determine the student's current level of oral reading skill through a CBM assessment. This is done by measuring the number of correctly read words versus errors a student makes in 1

Phonological Awareness: Initial Sound Generation

Directions:

Say, **I'm going to say a word. You tell me what sound the word starts with. Let's try one for practice.** *Ball.*
Ball **starts with /b/. Now you try one. What sound does _____ start with?**

Probe # __1_____

Item	Phonemes	Word	Student response
1	3	fad	/f/ Correct
2	2	be	/e/ Incorrect
3	3	log	/l/ Correct
4	4	cold	/c/ Correct
5	2	say	/s/ Correct
6	4	kept	/k/ Correct
7	3	pan	/d/ Incorrect
8	3	gas	/g/ Correct
9	3	was	/w/ Correct
10	4	trap	/ tr / Incorrect
11	2	it	/i/ Correct
12	4	tent	/t/ Correct
13	3	lid	/l/ Correct
14	3	top	/t/ Correct
15	4	left	/ / Incorrect (no response)
16	4	jump	/g/ Incorrect
17	2	so	/s/ Correct
18	3	pet	/p/ Correct
19	3	wish	/w/ Correct
20	4	tiger	/t/ Correct 1-minute mark here
21	3	fun	/f/ Correct
22	4	bump	/d/ Incorrect
23	2	up	/a/ Incorrect
24	4	gold	/g/ Correct
25	4	frog	/f/ Correct
26	3	tug	/t/ Correct
27	3	red	/l/ Incorrect
28	2	go	/g/ Correct
29	4	letter	/l/ Correct
30	4	press	/ / Incorrect (no response)

Accuracy = total correct / total administered = __21/30 70%__
Fluency = total correct per minute = __15__ (suggesting low accuracy and fluency)

FIGURE 3.1. Example of a scored initial segmentation probe.

Initial Screening

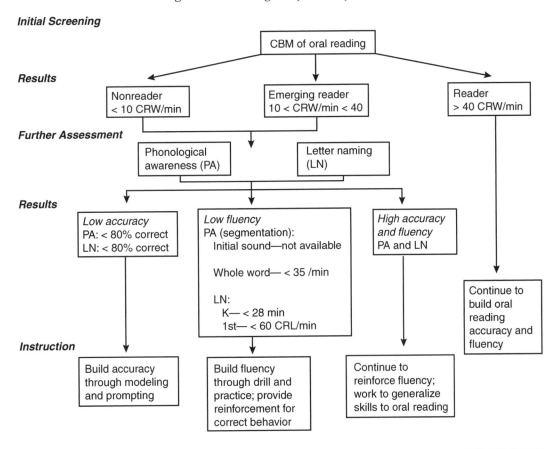

FIGURE 3.2. Early literacy assessment and intervention decision-making model. Information presented includes expectations for first-grade performance. Some of the information is based on research norms available from Good and Kaminski (2001).

minute while reading a passage taken from curriculum-level materials (described in Chapter 4). Many younger or lower-skilled students may perform poorly on a measure of oral reading skill. However, this initial step allows the establishment of baseline information regarding current student level of skill, which will then be useful when examining student response to various instructional strategies.

As a general guideline, Good and Kaminski (2001) have suggested that by the spring of first grade, established readers should be able to read orally more than 40 words correctly in 1 minute. According to Good and Kaminski's (2001) benchmarks, ideally a second-grade student at this same time should read at least 90 correct words per minute. As can be noted in the flowchart, reading between 10 and 40 words correctly per minute is classified as "emerging," whereas reading less than 10 is considered "nonreader." Further assessment is recommended for any student falling into these two categories; assessment should focus on the specific early literacy skills of letter-naming fluency and phonological awareness. As would be expected, a nonreader probably will need more intensive instruction, whereas an emerging reader may simply need some gaps filled in or additional support. In contrast, an established reader probably already possesses sufficient early literacy skills. Thus, instruction should focus on continuing to build reading accuracy and fluency.

Further information regarding selection of appropriate instructional packages can be found in the following section on intervention. When determining intervention, a primary goal is to evaluate the current instructional program within the context of the identified needs of the student being assessed. (Further information regarding the instructional environment can be found in Chapter 2.)

Case Example

John is a second-grade student who was described by his teacher as not keeping pace with his peers in reading. When his oral reading fluency was assessed in first-grade reading passages (his instructional level), John correctly read 29 words per minute (see Figure 3.3), placing him in the category of emerging reader. Further assessment of letter naming suggested that John is both accurate (94%) and fluent (72 correctly read letters per minute). Phonological awareness assessment revealed that John was able to accurately segment the sounds in a word (100% accuracy with the first sound) but did not do so rapidly (fluency of 30 correct segments per minute; Figure 3.3). Instructional recommendations included

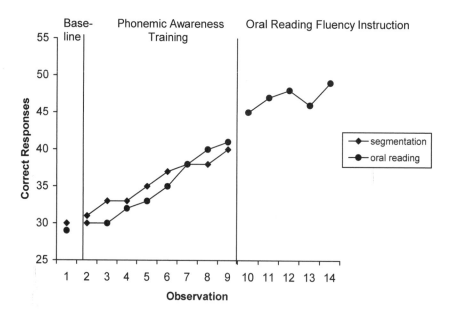

FIGURE 3.3. John's segmentation and oral reading fluency results. Baseline assessment establishes John as an "emerging" reader who needs to build fluency in segmentation and oral reading. An intervention package that included reading practice in controlled text and whole-word segmentation activities was implemented, until oral reading fluency measures indicated that John had become a "reader." Then segmentation assessment and instruction were dropped, and reading practice and oral reading fluency assessment were continued.

continued reading practice in controlled text, along with drill and practice and reinforcement for correct behavior in phonological awareness. Oral reading and phonological awareness skill (whole-word segmentation) continued to be assessed to monitor his performance. His progress is graphed in Figure 3.3.

HOW SHOULD WE PROVIDE EARLY LITERACY INTERVENTION?

Early literacy training studies have repeatedly suggested that instruction in both phonological awareness and letter–sound correspondences produce the largest, most enduring effects. For example, a 7-week intervention implemented by Ball and Blachman (1991) found that a group receiving instruction only in letter–sound correspondences made fewer gains in areas of early reading, spelling, and segmentation than a group who received a combination of phoneme segmentation and letter–sound correspondence training. Perhaps the most astounding finding in literacy training studies is the relatively small amount of training time needed to produce substantial benefits for many students. For example, in the Ball and Blachman (1991) study, students met in small groups for 15–20 minutes, four times per week, for 7 weeks. Given these consistent and impressive findings, the cost of allocating instructional time to early literacy instruction certainly seems minimal relative to the benefits that can be achieved.

Characteristics of a Good Intervention

Perhaps the most essential characteristic of good early literacy intervention is that it includes an *explicit approach* to instruction, in which sounds in letters are taught in isolation and then blended to form words, rather than, for example, simply stating a word and repeating the first sound. The initial focus is on mastering a few letter–sound correspondences so that words can then be read by putting those sounds together. In contrast, an *implicit approach* focuses on identification of letter sounds within the context of the whole word (Stein, Johnson, & Gutlohn, 1999). Context and picture cues are often used to read an unfamiliar word. For example, a teacher provides a clue to a word by saying another word that begins with the same sound and then asking the student to think of another word with the same sound that also fits in the sentence. In addition to an explicit approach to instruction, a number of other characteristics are associated with good early literacy instruction. A list of these characteristics, adapted from work compiled by Stahl et al. (1998), is presented in Table 3.4. Although all are important, specific attention should be paid to the idea that instruction should be stimulating, not boring. As stated earlier, explicit instruction for short periods may be all that is needed for most students, with the specific activities tailored to their developmental needs.

Early literacy can be developed most beneficially through early and direct teacher instruction in the specific skills of phonological awareness and letter knowledge. This instruction should be focused at a level that allows for high rates of successful student per-

TABLE 3.4. Principles of Good Early
Literacy Instruction

Good early literacy instruction should . . .
    Develop the alphabetic principle
    Develop phonological awareness
    Provide a thorough grounding in the letters
    Be stimulating, not boring
    Provide sufficient practice in reading words
    Lead to automatic word recognition

Note. Data from Stahl et al. (1998).

formance. To maximize success, the requirements of a task can be structured in various
ways to match the student's skill level. Some options for modifying phonological awareness tasks are highlighted in Table 3.5. For example, a segmentation task could involve
segmenting part of a word (easier) or segmenting the entire word (harder). In terms of
teaching letter knowledge, the overall goal is to develop automatic recognition; current
perspectives as to whether to teach letter names, letter sounds, or both, however, are not
consistent. Both Adams (1990) and Stahl et al. (1998) recommend teaching names and
sounds because (1) acquisition of letter names is a good predictor of further skills, and
(2) knowing names and sounds helps children talk about letters. To reiterate, it is important to recognize that the level of complexity varies both across and within early literacy
tasks. Although the ultimate goal is the ability to produce responses at the phonemic
level, initial instruction may focus on identification and then lead to production in order
to provide sufficient help to allow success. An example intervention protocol (adapted
from a study by Daly, Chafouleas, Persampieri, Bonfiglio, & Lafleur, 2004) for building
accuracy with blending and segmentation skills is presented in Figure 3.4. This protocol

TABLE 3.5. Variations for Teaching Phonological Awareness

Principle	Easier example	Harder example
Complexity varies within activities.	Does *sat* rhyme with *cat*?	What rhymes with *sat*?
Awareness at the syllable level is easier than the phonemic level.	/s/-at	/s/-/a/-/t/
Continuant phonemes are easier than noncontinuant.	/s/- a- t →	/p/-a-t →
Initial consonants are easier than final consonants.	*sat*—/s/	*sat*—/t/
Manipulatives (disks) can be helpful.		
Fewer phonemes are easier than more.	*sat*—three phonemes /s/-/a/-/t/	*saturn*—five phonemes /s/-/a/-/t/-/ur/-/n/

Note. Data from Catts (1995).

Materials Checklist:

Four flashcards of instructional words (choose words the student is unable to read, but which are decodable and whose letters have predictable and not unusual sounds).

Blank flashcard

Instructions for Administration:

1. Shuffle the instructional cards.
2. Say, "TODAY, WE ARE GOING TO LEARN HOW TO READ SOME WORDS AND THEN PRACTICE BREAKING THEM APART AND PUTTING THEM BACK TOGETHER. DO YOU HAVE ANY QUESTIONS?"
3. Present the **first flashcard**, covering the word with the blank flashcard. Say, "I WILL SHOW YOU SOUNDS IN THE WORD, TELL YOU THE SOUNDS, AND THEN HAVE YOU READ THE SOUNDS."
4. Expose the first phoneme by withdrawing the blank flashcard from it and say, "THE SOUND IS _____." Wait for a student response and say, "GOOD!" [If the student makes an error, say, "NO. THE SOUND IS _____. SAY THE SOUND. GOOD!"]. Repeat this step for all phonemes in the words, successively exposing each phoneme until the student can see the whole word.
5. Say, "LET'S SAY THE SOUNDS TOGETHER AS A WORD. SAY THEM TOGETHER REAL FAST. THE WORD IS _____."
6. Repeat steps 3, 4, and 5 for the **second flashcard**.
7. Repeat steps 3, 4, and 5 for the **third flashcard**.
8. Repeat steps 3, 4, and 5 for the **fourth flashcard**.
9. Shuffle the instructional cards.
10. Say, "NOW, I WANT YOU TO READ THE SOUNDS AND WORDS TO ME. IF YOU ARE NOT SURE OF A SOUND OR WORD, I WILL HELP YOU."
11. Present a flashcard to the student, exposing one phoneme at a time. If the student does not read a phoneme within **3** seconds, say the phoneme for the student and have the student repeat the sound (saying "REPEAT AFTER ME!" if the student does not repeat the sound spontaneously).
12. At the end of the word, say, "SAY THE SOUNDS TOGETHER AS A WORD. SAY THEM TOGETHER REAL FAST."
13. Repeat steps 11 and 12 for the **second flashcard**.
14. Repeat steps 11 and 12 for the **third flashcard**.
15. Repeat steps 11 and 12 for the **fourth flashcard**.
16. Shuffle the instructional cards.
17. Say, "LET'S PRACTICE ONE LAST TIME."
18. Repeat steps 11 and 12 once more for each word.
19. Shuffle the instructional cards and say, "NOW I WILL SHOW YOU THE CARDS AGAIN AND I WANT YOU TO READ THE WHOLE WORD TO ME." (Provide correction and have the student repeat correct responses, if needed.)

FIGURE 3.4. Example of an instructional lesson for building accuracy with blending and segmentation skills.

can be modified to address fluency or motivation issues by including, for example, a reward component for correctly read words, or through timing and tracking speed of item completion as a part of an assessment that could be done either at the beginning or end of the instructional session.

Selecting an Intervention

Although further systematic research is needed to evaluate existing reading programs and identify "best" options, the most effective programs currently available include "early and systematic" effort in improving the very skills discussed in this chapter (Stahl et al., 1998). In addition, we would emphasize that it is not essential to use a prepackaged program. Rather, adherence to general principles of good early literacy instruction, such as those presented in the chapter, coupled with good assessment and decision making form the basis for successful acquisition of early literacy skills. (However, there *are* some good prepackaged programs available; see Appendix 3.1 at the end of the chapter.) A form for evaluating instructional tools can be found on Worksheet 3.4.

Return for a moment to the flowchart presented in Figure 3.2. This flowchart helps direct you to the area in need of intervention, based on the results of the assessment. Instructional intervention should be framed around a clear identification of the student's skill level. For example, if assessment reveals that a student has low phonological awareness accuracy, then instructional goals would include building accuracy through strategies such as modeling and prompting. Enhancing phonological awareness could involve implementation of an activity such as Say It and Move It (described below). Table 3.6 outlines the principles of instruction for each stage along with some specific activity ideas. Procedures for some of those activities are provided next.

Having outlined some core requirements of intervention selection, we now provide a description of, and materials for, a simple early literacy instructional program. The instructional components selected are based on work by Blachman and colleagues and are clearly described in the seminal study conducted by Ball and Blachman (1991).

TABLE 3.6. Instructional Activities Appropriate for Each Level of Student Proficiency

Instructional stage	Instructional principles	Examples	Worksheet
Acquisition (accuracy)	Modeling	Say It and Move It	3.5a–d
	Prompting	Letter cards	3.5a–d
Fluency	Drill and practice	Sound bingo	3.7a–f
	Reinforcement of correct behavior	Rewarding performance increases	
Generalization		Reading in controlled text	
		Other PA activities	

The early literacy instructional program created by Ball and Blachman (1991) is composed of three separate activities that are implemented approximately 15 minutes per day. Instruction is presented in small groups whose composition is determined by instructional skill level. Two of the activities—one emphasizing phonological awareness (Say It and Move It) and the other, letter–sound correspondences—remain consistent across sessions, whereas the third activity reinforces phonological awareness through various fun activities. It is recommended that only a few letters be selected initially for focus, and that words used within activities be sequenced by difficulty, such as beginning with two-phoneme words and then perhaps adding CVC (consonant–vowel–consonant) words. There are no hard-and-fast rules for selection of the specific letters for focus. However, due to their utility for use in monosyllabic words, Adams, Foorman, Lundberg, and Beeler (1998) suggest starting with short vowels (*a, e, i, o, u*) and the following consonants: s, m, d, p, t, n, g, b, r, f, l.

Descriptions of each of the three separate activities follow:

1. *Say It and Move It.* In this segmentation activity, the student is taught to represent each sound with a manipulative (e.g., disk, checker, letter). A sheet (can be laminated for durability) is provided that has a picture of a place to "hold" the disks; below it are boxes, the number of which corresponds to the number of phonemes in the presented word (two, three, or four). Directions can be found on Worksheet 3.5a and reproducible examples on Worksheets 3.5b–d. The presentation of an item to segment follows a sequence in which the teacher models and then the student responds in the same manner. The student is taught to move one manipulative (i.e., disk) into each box, from left to right, while slowly pronouncing the sound represented. Once a student masters the concept of moving a manipulative into the box while stating the sound, segmenting with two-phoneme words and then three-phoneme words can be introduced.

2. *Letter–sound correspondences.* Teaching letter–sound correspondences includes strategies involving keywords and phrases. For example, composing jingles to illustrate letters (*A: ants ate apples*) is one fun way to reinforce letter–sound correspondences. Letter cards can be found in Worksheet 3.6a–d. In addition, games such as bingo can be modified to use sounds and letters (see Sound Bingo, Worksheets 3.7a–f). As a final example, the program outlined in Blachman, Ball, Black, and Tangel (2000) describes a game titled "Post Office." In this activity, students "mail" letters or pictures into the appropriate pouches. Letters replace the other manipulatives after several letter–sound correspondences are mastered.

3. *Phonological awareness.* The final part of each lesson engages students in another phonological awareness activity, which can vary from lesson to lesson. Examples of other activities include sound blending using puppets, counting the number of phonemes in words, and categorizing them based on common rhymes and sounds. This activity reinforces generalization of learned skills across materials and activities.

A final word on selection of materials, specifically, the need for "decodable" text, is in order. Although early literacy instruction can be provided within the use of existing classroom materials, some attention to the selection of reading materials should be given. Selected materials should emphasize the specific skills taught in the early literacy instruction so that students have ample opportunity to practice applying the skills that have been newly acquired. For example, if the short vowel *a* has been taught, then materials involving the short vowel *a* would be beneficial. This method is known as providing decodable text to the student. An examination of major first-grade basal reading programs, conducted by Stein and colleagues (1999), noted that those programs with a high proportion of decodable text also emphasized an explicit approach to teacher instruction. The bad news is that only one of seven basal student readers (i.e., Open Court's *Collections for Young Scholars*, 1995) contained a sufficient percentage of decodable words (≥ 50%). The implication of this finding is that you may need to spend time sampling various curriculum materials or real texts in order to find appropriate decodable reading materials. For example, Stein et al. (1999) suggest taking random selections of text and separating the words into lists of (1) decodable, (2) sight, and (3) nondecodable/noninstructed words (specific directions for completing such an analysis can be found in the Curriculum Evaluation Worksheet provided in the Stein et al. article). Although guidelines for determining appropriate proportions vary depending on intended use, Beck (1997) recommended that text read by students early in first grade should be 70–80% decodable.

How Do I Know If the Intervention Is Working?

Once the area of weakness has been initially identified and an instructional intervention has been recommended, it is important to continue assessment of the weakness on a repeated basis. In addition, it may be appropriate to assess progress in long-term goal areas, such as oral reading. For example, in the case described above, John was identified as an emerging reader and as needing to build fluency in phonological awareness. Progress monitoring for him may include the area of phonological awareness (short-term goal of phonological awareness fluency) as well as CBM for oral reading (long-term goal of reading fluency). Progress monitoring facilitates informed decision making regarding the effectiveness of the intervention and improves the quality of decisions about whether the intervention should continue as is, be modified, or changed altogether. Worksheet 3.8 provides a summary sheet that can be used to record progress-monitoring information. These data can be plotted on a graph to make it possible to assess trends over time.

Case Example

Returning to John, our emerging reader (Figure 3.3), we note that he had mastered letter naming but was not yet able to segment whole words fluently. Thus, instructional recommendations included continued reading practice in controlled text along with drill and practice and reinforcement for correct segmenting and blending. Because John is a second-grade student and had demonstrated mastery of letter–sound correspondences, it was decided that a modified Say It and Move It activity would be implemented as the primary phonological awareness intervention. During this activity, John used letters as the manipulatives, and the activity was structured as a speed game. That is, John was told to segment as many whole words as he could in 1 minute and to chart his correct segments on a daily basis. Error correction was provided for each mistake, and John received praise and small tangibles (stickers for his chart) for correct performance. John continued to participate in the regular reading curriculum, reading trade books and curriculum materials that appropriately matched his instructional level. Progress monitoring in phonological awareness (whole-word segmentation) and oral reading was continued twice a week; his progress appears in Figure 3.3. Phonological awareness assessment was discontinued once oral reading fluency was established.

SUMMARY

This chapter focused on the important role of early literacy skills as the building blocks of future reading success. Two discrete early literacy skills, phonological awareness and letter knowledge, were highlighted, based on the substantial literature base supporting the critical role these skills play in understanding the alphabetic principle, which is a crucial accomplishment on the way to accurate and fluent reading of text. An assessment and intervention framework was presented to guide informed decision making that maximizes progress toward fluent reading. Assessment and intervention materials to implement the decision-making framework were provided and resources for finding and evaluating additional materials were suggested.

APPENDIX 3.1. Additional Early Literacy Intervention Package Resources

WHOLE-CLASS INSTRUCTION

Phonemic Awareness in Young Children (Adams, Foorman, Lundberg, & Beeler, 1998)

Ladders to Literacy, Preschool Activity Book (Notari-Syverson, O'Connor, & Vadasy, 1998)

Ladders to Literacy, Kindergarten Activity Book (O'Connor, Notari-Syverson, & Vadasy, 1998)

Available from: Brookes Publishing Company, *www.brookespublishing.com*, 800-638-3775.

SMALL-GROUP INSTRUCTION

Road to the Code: A Phonological Awareness Program for Young Children (Blachman, Ball, Black, & Tangel, 2000)

Available from: Brookes Publishing Company, *www.brookespublishing.com*, 800-638-3775.

Phonological Awareness Training for Reading (Torgesen & Bryant, 1994b)

The Lindamood Phoneme Sequencing Program for Reading, Spelling, and Speech (formerly known as *Auditory Discrimination in Depth*) (Lindamood & Lindamood, 1998)

Available from: PRO-ED, Inc., *http://www.proedinc.com/index.html*, 800-897-3202.

COMPUTER SOFTWARE

The Learning Company; *www.broderbund.com*, 800-395-0277.

WORKSHEET 3.1. Evaluating Assessment Tools

Title of Measure: _____

Skills Assessed: _____

Age Range: _____

Administration Time: _____

Scores Available: _____

	Low				High
What evidence of reliability is available?	1	2	3	4	5

What is the range of scores?
Does the test require production or selection response?
What types of reliability information are provided (e.g.,
alternate form, test–retest)?

	Low				High
What evidence of validity is available?	1	2	3	4	5

Does the test measure what it is supposed to measure?
Is it predictive of future reading achievement?
Can the test be used repeatedly? (i.e., multiple alternate
forms available)

	Not at all			Definitely	
To what degree will the information gained from the test easily inform instructional intervention?	1	2	3	4	5
Do the items reflect an appropriate difficulty level?	1	2	3	4	5
If the intent is to use the measure with multiple students, is it feasible to administer and manage the data?	1	2	3	4	5

	No				Yes
Is this measure appropriate for this (these) student(s)?					

WORKSHEET 3.2a. Directions for Administering and Scoring Letter Naming

Materials:

Letter-naming probe sheet for student
Letter-naming probe sheet for teacher
Stopwatch

Directions:

Say, **I am going to show you a page with some letters on it. When I say** *begin*, **I want you to say the names of each of the letters out loud. Read across the page like this.** Demonstrate with your finger how to read the words from the child's left to right. **When you finish the first row, go on to the next row and keep reading.** Again, point out with finger. **If you get to the end of the page before I say stop, turn the page and keep reading. If you get to a letter that you don't know, I will tell you its name. Do the best you can. Do you have any questions?**

Say *begin*, and start the stopwatch when the student says the first letter. If the student hesitates for more than 3 seconds on the first letter, say the name of the letter and start the stopwatch. If the student hesitates for more than 3 seconds on any letter, read the name of that letter aloud. At the end of 1 minute, say **stop**. Make a bracket ( ]) after the last letter read on your sheet to indicate the last letter read or attempted.

Scoring:

Correct pronunciations and self-corrections are scored as correct. Mispronunciations, omissions, and hesitations of more than 3 seconds are scored as incorrect.
Accuracy Scoring = total correct / total administered = _____%
Fluency Scoring = total correct before bracket = _____/min

WORKSHEET 3.2b. Letter-Naming Probes

K	U	T	J	M
O	E	R	B	P
Y	F	A	Z	N
H	D	W	Q	G
X	C	L	S	V
W	H	A	D	R
I	K	E	J	S
T	U	C	V	X
O	Y	F	M	L
B	Q	P	G	N
Z	B	Y	O	T
J	S	F	E	K

A	Q	X	K	F
D	W	R	V	U
H	P	E	J	T
C	S	L	M	B
O	Y	Z	N	H
G	F	H	X	U
V	W	Z	Q	Y
N	R	O	M	P
K	D	L	J	A
I	E	B	S	C
G	T	K	R	Z
Y	A	S	M	I

WORKSHEET 3.2d. Letter-Naming Probes

G	B	Y	P	O
I	D	R	X	E
F	H	U	M	K
J	W	Q	S	L
C	A	G	T	V
Z	N	E	S	L
D	F	R	O	I
K	X	W	G	P
Q	V	B	N	J
H	N	A	E	U
C	T	M	Z	A
D	W	P	S	D

WORKSHEET 3.2e. Letter-Naming Probes

E	G	P	Z	Y
N	I	A	X	J
W	S	K	B	U
D	O	H	V	L
T	F	Q	C	R
M	C	P	R	E
Z	M	D	H	C
V	G	F	O	Y
W	J	Q	L	N
U	X	K	S	T
B	A	I	C	D
S	W	P	M	H

WORKSHEET 3.2f. Letter-Naming Probes

C	U	J	G	T
H	B	M	Q	K
D	F	I	W	N
O	P	V	R	X
Z	S	J	Y	L
A	E	T	K	D
C	R	O	I	P
W	U	S	L	G
F	A	X	H	Y
B	M	E	V	Q
N	Z	T	R	L
P	O	M	U	K

WORKSHEET 3.3a. Phonological Awareness: Initial Sound Segmentation

Directions:

Say, **I'm going to say a word. You tell me what sound the word starts with. Let's try one for practice.** *Ball. Ball* **starts with /b/. Now you try one. What sound does _____ start with?** (Select words from columns on Worksheet 3.3c.)

Probe # _____

Item	Phonemes	Word	Student response
1	3		/ /
2	2		/ /
3	3		/ /
4	4		/ /
5	2		/ /
6	4		/ /
7	3		/ /
8	3		/ /
9	3		/ /
10	4		/ /
11	2		/ /
12	4		/ /
13	3		/ /
14	3		/ /
15	4		/ /
16	4		/ /
17	2		/ /
18	3		/ /
19	3		/ /
20	4		/ /

(continued)

Phonological Awareness: Initial Sound Segmentation *(page 2 of 2)*

Item	Phonemes	Word	Student response
21	3		/ /
22	4		/ /
23	2		/ /
24	4		/ /
25	4		/ /
26	3		/ /
27	3		/ /
28	2		/ /
29	4		/ /
30	4		/ /

Accuracy = total correct / total administered = _____%

Fluency = total correct per minute = _____

WORKSHEET 3.3b. Phonological Awareness: Whole-Word Segmentation

Directions:

Give the child five manipulatives (e.g., disks). Say, **I'm going to say a word. You tell me how many sounds you hear in the word. Say each sound and move one disk for each sound that you say. Let's try one for practice. The word is** *it*. *It* **has two sounds, /i/ /t/. Move one disk for each sound that you say. Now, it's your turn. How many sounds does the word** _____ **have?** (Select words from columns on Worksheet 3.3c.)

Probe # _____

Item	Phonemes	Word	Student response
1	3		/ / / / / / / /
2	2		/ / / / / / / /
3	3		/ / / / / / / /
4	4		/ / / / / / / /
5	2		/ / / / / / / /
6	4		/ / / / / / / /
7	3		/ / / / / / / /
8	3		/ / / / / / / /
9	3		/ / / / / / / /
10	4		/ / / / / / / /
11	2		/ / / / / / / /
12	4		/ / / / / / / /
13	3		/ / / / / / / /
14	3		/ / / / / / / /
15	4		/ / / / / / / /
16	4		/ / / / / / / /
17	2		/ / / / / / / /
18	3		/ / / / / / / /
19	3		/ / / / / / / /
20	4		/ / / / / / / /

(continued)

Phonological Awareness: Whole-Word Segmentation *(page 2 of 2)*

Item	Phonemes	Word	Student response
21	3		/ / / / / / / /
22	4		/ / / / / / / /
23	2		/ / / / / / / /
24	4		/ / / / / / / /
25	4		/ / / / / / / /
26	3		/ / / / / / / /
27	3		/ / / / / / / /
28	2		/ / / / / / / /
29	4		/ / / / / / / /
30	4		/ / / / / / / /

Accuracy = total correct segments / total administered = _____%

Fluency = total correct per minute = _____

WORKSHEET 3.3c. Phonological Awareness Assessment: Word Selection Grid

Directions:

Use the words from this chart to create phonological awareness tasks on Worksheets 3.3a and 3.3b. Randomly select words from the category corresponding to the number of phonemes, until the entire probe sheet is completed.

	Initial sound	
	Continuant	Noncontinuant
Two-phoneme words	at age all as eat ice in it of out row say so up	be boy by day die do dough go tea toe to toy
Three-phoneme words	fad fan fat fed fin fit fun lag led leg let lid lip log lot rag ran rat red rig rim rip rod rot rug rum sad sat set sin sit sip sod sum sun was wet will wish yes	bag bat bed big bit bug but cap cat can cup dad den dig dip dog dug gas gun jam jet jog job jug kid kin pan pet pin pig pot pup tab tag tap ten tin top tug
Four-phoneme words	city fact fast felt film flag flop fork found frog into land last lazy left letter lump open rest round sand sent scan short sick silk silly skip slid smog snag soft swim spell stem step want weld wind yarn	baby bank belt best black blot brass bump bunny busy camp cart cast class clap crib cold dark drop gasp gold grin gust jump just kept kind pant pest pond pizza plan press prop tent tiger tiny trap truck twig

WORKSHEET 3.4. Evaluating Instructional Tools

Title of intervention: _____

Skills taught: _____

_____

_____

Session length: _____

Intervention program length, if applicable: _____

Does the intervention include explicit instruction? *Example:*	No				Yes

Does the intervention emphasize an opportunity for modeling?	Never 1	2	3	Frequently 4	5
Does the intervention emphasize an opportunity for feedback?	Never 1	2	3	Frequently 4	5
Does the intervention emphasize an opportunity for practice?	Never 1	2	3	Frequently 4	5
Are the materials appropriate (i.e., interesting) for the intended student(s)?	Not at all 1	2	3	4	Highly 5
Are resources needed to implement procedures readily available in the setting?	None 1	2	3	4	All 5

Comments:

_____

_____

_____

Is this intervention appropriate?	No		Yes

WORKSHEET 3.5a. Directions for Say It and Move It

Materials:

One Say-It-and-Move-It worksheet per child
Two to four manipulatives per child (disks, checkers, or letters)

Directions:

Give each child a Say-It-and-Move-It worksheet and the appropriate number of manipulatives. Place the manipulatives on the picture of the treasure chest (Worksheets 3.5b, 3.5c, or 3.5d, depending on number of phonemes being studied).

TEACHER: **Watch me and listen. I'm going to say a word.** [*Insert word here.*]

TEACHER: **Now I am going to say it and move it.** Place your fingers on the manipulative and hold out the first sound while you move one manipulative from the treasure chest to the further left box at the bottom of the sheet. Then quickly move the second manipulative to the next box while saying the next sound in the word. Repeat until all sounds in the word have been pronounced.

TEACHER: [*Insert word here.*] *Repeat the word while moving your finger from left to right under the manipulatives.*

TEACHER: **Now it's your turn. Say** [*insert word here.*] Wait for response.

TEACHER: **Now say it and move it.**

WORKSHEET 3.5b. Two-Phoneme Card for Say It and Move It

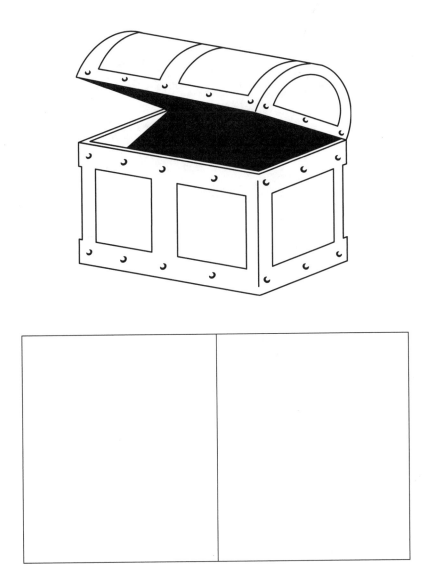

WORKSHEET 3.5c. Three-Phoneme Card for Say It and Move It

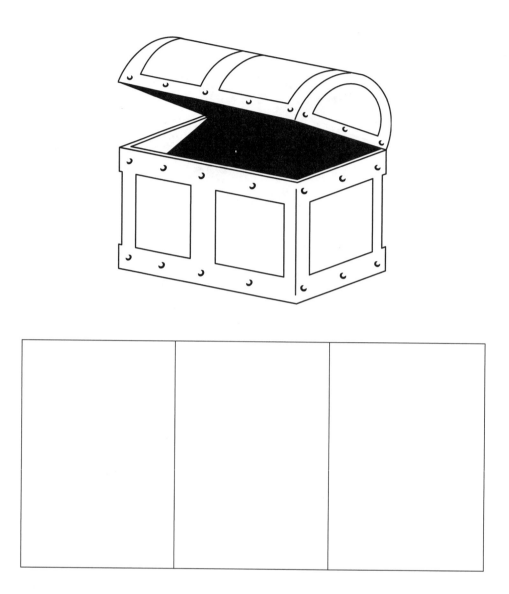

WORKSHEET 3.5d. Four-Phoneme Card for Say It and Move It

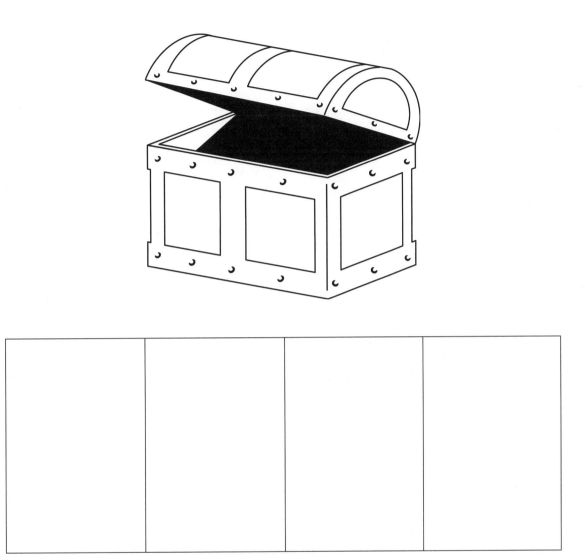

a	b
c	d
e	f
g	h

WORKSHEET 3.6b. Letter Cards

i	j
k	l
m	n

WORKSHEET 3.6c. Letter Cards

o	p
q	r
s	t

u	v
w	x
y	z

WORKSHEET 3.7a. Directions for Sound Bingo

Materials:

One sound bingo card per child
Several bingo chips per child

Directions:

Make copies of the picture and letter squares (Worksheets 3.7b and 3.7c). Place these squares into a box or bag. To play, draw out one square at a time and show it to the students. If a picture square is drawn, the students should name the picture and give the first sound. Any student who has that picture on his or her cards should place a bingo chip on it. If a letter square is drawn, the students should give the sound of that letter. Any student who has that letter on his or her cards should place a bingo chip on it. The teacher can decide in advance whether the students need to cover a single row or the entire card to get "bingo."

WORKSHEET 3.7b. Sound Bingo Card: Letter Squares

S	M	T
D	P	N
G	B	R
C	L	F
H	J	W

WORKSHEET 3.7c. Sound Bingo Card: Picture Squares

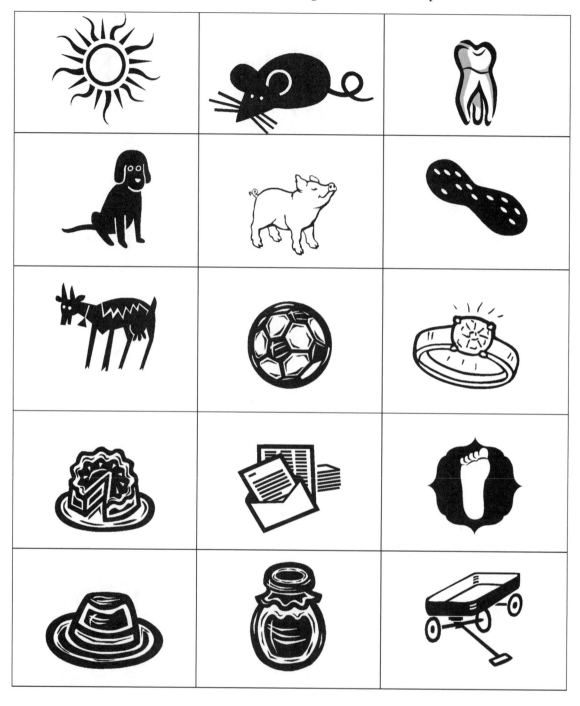

S		W
	T	
H		J
		D

M		C
R		
	T	
	L	W

G	F	
	N	P
T		B

WORKSHEET 3.8. Progress Monitoring Summary Sheet

Student Name: _____

Grade/Class: _____

Initial Assessment Results and Recommendations

Date	Area(s) of assessment	Results		Instructional Plan
		Accuracy	Fluency	
_____	_____	_____	_____	_____
_____	_____	_____	_____	_____

Progress Monitoring Information

Date	Area(s) of assessment	Results		Instructional Plan
		Accuracy	Fluency	
_____	_____	_____	_____	_____
_____	_____	_____	_____	_____
_____	_____	_____	_____	_____
_____	_____	_____	_____	_____
_____	_____	_____	_____	_____
_____	_____	_____	_____	_____
_____	_____	_____	_____	_____
_____	_____	_____	_____	_____
_____	_____	_____	_____	_____
_____	_____	_____	_____	_____
_____	_____	_____	_____	_____
_____	_____	_____	_____	_____
_____	_____	_____	_____	_____
_____	_____	_____	_____	_____

4

Producing Measurable Increases in Reading Fluency

The majority of educational programs and curricula overwhelmingly emphasize accuracy (e.g., 80% correct) on tasks such as book tests and end-of-chapter tests. Teachers often rely on this information for decisions about whether to move students further along in the curriculum or not. Although being accurate is important, if a student is to be expected to progress to harder materials and subjects, an equally important criterion is how quickly he or she responds when asked to perform "on demand" or do an assignment. This issue is particularly important in the area of reading, where students learn to read so that they can ultimately read to learn. Reading must become fluid and efficient if it is to be useful and, hopefully, even pleasurable for the student. Developing reading fluency is an important step to becoming a competent reader, because it increases the student's capacity to use reading as a helpful tool (and not an added burden) with more difficult tasks. It is therefore a legitimate target for instruction and remediation. Many reading problems are fluency problems (which include both accurate and rapid word reading). Only a small percentage of reading problems concern problems with comprehension. Of course, poor reading fluency is likely to lead to poor comprehension as well, and it may hinder students' motivation to tackle more complicated tasks, such as those associated with research papers and such.

This chapter provides a rationale for enhancing speed of accurate, oral reading. Procedures for assessing reading fluency are described, as are strategies designed to enhance it. A variety of empirically validated intervention strategies are described in sufficient detail to get you started. We present each strategy individually, with a rationale for appropriate use, so that you can assemble just the right components to create an intervention tailored to the circumstances of the referral problem. For instance, if you are starting a tutoring program and will be using the intervention with a group of students, a procedurally simpler intervention is probably preferable; you might prioritize a smaller set of strategies. If, however, you are working with a single student who is having severe and persistent difficulties, you probably would want a stronger treatment and would therefore combine more intervention components. The chapter concludes with a description of how these strategies can be embedded in various tutoring and instructional formats, including a description of classwide peer tutoring.

WHY IS FLUENCY IMPORTANT?

Reading fluency is defined operationally as the number of correctly read words per minute when an individual is asked to read a passage of connected text aloud for 1 minute. We address the details of administration and scoring later. Here we wish to point out that this simple measure has helped to explain a lot of things about the process of reading acquisition, in general, and about why some readers struggle, in particular. Research on reading fluency has been quite productive, even if there have been differing explanations for why fluency is important. We can readily identify three reasons why you should consider this factor to be a critical and legitimate intervention target (see Table 4.1). Each reason is discussed below.

Fluent Readers Are More Likely to Comprehend

Fluency is a strong indicator of overall reading competence (Shinn, 1989), and measured fluency is superior to comprehension measures for younger students (Shinn, Good, Knutson, & Tilly, 1992). Furthermore, correlations between reading fluency and reading comprehension are strong (Hintze, Callahan, Matthews, Williams, & Tobin, 2002; Kranzler, Brownell, & Miller, 1998; Marston, 1989; Shinn et al., 1992). Although not sufficient alone for comprehension, fluency is a necessary condition for adequate independent comprehension.

There are a couple of ways to look at how fluency affects comprehension. First, the sequence and configuration of letters forming words on the page control your reading

---

TABLE 4.1. What the Research Says about
Why Reading Fluency Is Important

1. Fluent readers are more likely to comprehend what they are reading.

2. Building fluency is likely to make reading a more rewarding experience and may increase the chances that a student will actually *choose* to read rather than choose to do other things.

3. Building fluency makes reading less effortful and therefore less frustrating for students—factors that also increase the chances that a student might actually choose to read rather than do other things.

when words are correctly read. You can't just make up what you want to read on the page! Interestingly, poor readers tend to overemphasize cues that are not textual (e.g., relying on pictures), to the detriment of their reading, whereas good readers have been shown to attend to virtually every letter on the page (Adams, 1990). When a learner becomes fluent with reading words in texts, the action of reading the word on the page competes more effectively with wrong responses such as making an incorrect guess about a word, waiting for someone to say the word, or looking around. When the reader is fluent, word reading is strong and durable across a variety of texts. As such, correctly reading the word is the most likely response when the word appears in print in the text. This textual control also makes it more likely that the reader will use the previously learned words as a basis for answering comprehension questions when queried by a teacher or parent about what the text is saying. Fluent readers are more likely to generalize to harder tasks such as answering comprehension questions, because their word reading is more strongly connected to the text at the very outset.

An alternate viewpoint is that readers who read accurately but slowly expend a lot of energy attempting to decode words and therefore have a lowered capacity to comprehend while they are reading (LaBerge & Samuels, 1974; Perfetti, 1977; Samuels, 1987). Furthermore, it is harder for less fluent readers to relate information presented earlier to material being currently read, as they work their way through a long text, because the ability to retain information tends to decay over time (Daneman & Carpenter, 1980; Samuels, 1987). A faster reader is more likely to access information presented earlier because the information has had less time to decay.

At one time or another, most of us have experienced problems with accessing information read earlier. For example, imagine Joe, who is lying in his hammock on a nice summer's day, reading a mystery novel for pleasure. While reading he is interrupted when a neighbor's dog unexpectedly arrives and begins barking. Joe, being a good neighbor, marks his place, puts his book down, and spends the next 20 minutes chasing the neighbor's dog. After finally securing the dog and returning him to his neighbor, Joe settles back into his hammock, opens the book to his mark, and begins reading exactly where he left off. Unfortunately, what he is reading makes little sense anymore. Joe does not even know with whom the main character is talking. These comprehension problems are caused by an inability to relate what he is currently reading to what he previously read. Joe remedies this problem by scanning back about four paragraphs and finding where this new person was introduced. As he rereads these paragraphs (getting a running start, so to speak), it comes back to him and the material once again makes sense. Now Joe can comprehend the material he is currently reading because he has accessed material presented earlier. Because he can now understand what he is reading, he once again begins to enjoy reading his novel.

Fluent Readers Are More Likely to Choose to Read

Those who read accurately but slowly may be less likely to choose to read than those who read fluently (Skinner, 1998). One factor that influences what a person chooses to do is how rewarding the experience is. In general, when faced with a choice between two or more actions, with all other factors held constant, people are more likely to choose to engage in actions that are more rewarding (Mace, McCurdy, & Quigley, 1990). To relate this principle to the reading process, suppose two students can both read the same material and comprehend 10 pieces of information. However, one student requires 10 minutes to read the material whereas the other requires 30 minutes. The student who reads the material in 10 minutes gains one piece of information for every minute spent reading. In contrast, the student who requires 30 minutes obtains only 1 piece of information for every 3 minutes of reading. Assuming that obtaining this information is rewarding in some way (e.g., heightened interest as a result of learning important clues in a mystery novel), the more rapid reader is being rewarded at three times the rate of the less fluent reader. Thus, the rapid reader may be more likely to choose to read than the slow reader, who may find rewards in doing other things. It turns out that slow readers may actually obtain *less* information (e.g., they may have difficulty relating information across materials, thus hindering comprehension). Furthermore, whereas strong readers may enjoy a beautifully written piece of work (e.g., finding that the flow of the language was "intoxicating"), slow readers may not be able to appreciate such well-written work because they cannot read rapidly enough to catch the nuances. For example, a beautifully written sentence may be difficult to appreciate when each word must be sounded out laboriously. Dysfluent readers may expend so much energy on decoding and comprehension that they are incapable of understanding subtle nuances that make reading a rewarding experience for others.

Fluent Reading Is Less Effortful

Slow readers may be less likely to choose to read than rapid readers because of the sheer effort involved when a skill is not proficiently employed. The effort slow readers must expend to comprehend written materials may make it less likely that they will choose to read assigned materials when there are alternative means of obtaining the information (Mace, Neef, Shade, & Mauro, 1996). For example, a dysfluent reader may be less likely to choose to read material that was assigned for homework and instead rely on class lecture to assist him or her in comprehending it, willingly settling for a lower grade. Even when they are not expected to learn information from text, slow readers are less likely to choose to read for pleasure because the amount of enjoyment they receive from reading may not be worth the high levels of effort that are required for them to read (Skinner, 1998).

ASSESSING READING FLUENCY USING CBM

Why Conduct Oral Reading Fluency Assessments?

As noted earlier, reading fluency can be assessed simply by having a student read a passage and recording correctly read words and errors during the first minute of reading. Curriculum-based measurement (CBM) is a standardized format for assessing reading fluency; it is so named because performance measures are generally based on curricular materials. Strong reliability and validity data support the use of CBM for decision making about students' reading proficiency and for a variety of common educational areas (Shinn, 1989, 1998). Oral reading fluency is a sensitive indicator of growth and instructional effects (Fuchs, Fuchs, Hamlett, Walz, & Germann, 1993).

Another advantage of CBM is that it is a low-budget and easy method for collecting high-quality information prior to and during interventions. However, you will need to put some thought into the purpose of the assessment and the selection of materials. Preparation of materials can cost you either time or money, depending on whether you want to make up reading probes (i.e., passages prepared for reading fluency assessments) or to purchase them. Finally, practicing the administration and scoring procedures is critical to accuracy, so a time investment is needed to learn how to administer and score reading fluency assessments. With initial assessments, we strongly advise checking your scoring against other people's scoring before considering the results "official." Directions for administration and scoring are standardized and can be found in Figure 4.1 Administration and scoring are not especially difficult. (To observe an oral reading fluency administration, go to *http://dibels.uoregon.edu/measures/orf.php* and click on the link for the video clip.) Once you have your assessment data, you can use Worksheet 4.1 (all worksheets are at the end of the chapter) to record the results. (This form is downloadable from the *interventioncentral.org* website.)

These administration and scoring procedures are at the heart of accomplishing the three purposes for CBM presented in this chapter: (1) identifying relative difficulty of current level (grade) of instructional materials, (2) gauging short-term growth as a result of reading interventions, and (3) gauging long-term growth in response to reading intervention. Depending on your purpose(s) for assessing, you will vary the probes/materials (including the number of probes administered in an assessment session) and the frequency with which you give the probes. (Further elaboration of each of these purposes is provided later in this chapter.) We turn now to the issue of choosing and preparing materials.

Reading Fluency Probes

First we consider general guidelines for selecting appropriate passages for reading fluency assessments, then we give specific directions for how to select materials. General guidelines for choosing CBM passages can be found in Worksheet 4.2. Although CBM probes can be taken directly from a student's reading curricular series, not all material in a series is appropriate for these probes. During CBM, a student's rate of accurate oral reading is being measured. However, some materials do not lend themselves to fluent reading. For example, poems, plays, and any material with a lot of dialogue, and material with many headings and subheadings, do not lend themselves to continuous, fluent reading. Instead, choose texts with continuous paragraphs.

Many current reading series are constructed to expose students to a variety of cultures and therefore include a variety of foreign words and names. It is unlikely that students will have had previous exposure to many of these words, and learned decoding skills may not be applicable. Therefore, these passages should be excluded when selecting and developing placement probes.

SPECIFIC DIRECTIONS FOR READING

Setting of Data Collection

The reading measures must be administered to students individually. Prepare two copies of each passage: a numbered copy for examiner use and an unnumbered copy for the student to read. You will need a stopwatch to keep track of time.

Directions

Say to the student: **When I say "start," begin reading aloud at the top of this page. Read across the page.** Demonstrate by pointing. **Try to read each word. If you come to a word you don't know, I'll tell it to you. Be sure to do your best reading. Are there any questions?**
Say **Start.**
Start your stopwatch when the student reads the first words and follow along on your copy of the story, marking the words that are read incorrectly. If the student stops or struggles with a word for 3 seconds, tell him or her the word and mark it as incorrect.
Place a bracket ( ]) after the last word read when 1 minute elapses. Have the student stop reading when it is convenient (e.g., at the end of the sentence) and thank him or her.
Count the number of words read correctly and incorrectly.

Scoring

The most important piece of information is the number of words read correctly. Reading fluency is a combination of speed and accuracy.

1. *Words read correctly.* Words read correctly are those words that are pronounced correctly, given the reading context.
   a. The word *read* must be pronounced *reed*, not as *red*, when the context is present or future tense (e.g., "He will read the book").
   b. Repetitions are not counted as incorrect.
   c. Self-corrections within 3 seconds are counted as correctly read words.
2. *Words read incorrectly.* The following types of errors are counted: (a) mispronunciations, (b) substitutions, and (c) omissions. In addition, words not read within 3 seconds are counted as errors.
   a. *Mispronunciations* are words that are misread: *dog* for *dig*.
   b. *Substitutions* are words that are substituted for the stimulus word; this is often inferred by a one-to-one correspondence between word order: *dog* for *cat*.
   c. *Omissions* are words skipped or not read; if a student skips an entire line, it is counted as one error only.*
3. *Three-second rule.* If a student is struggling to pronounce a word or hesitates for 3 seconds, the student is told the word, and it is counted as an error.

FIGURE 4.1. Directions for curriculum-based measurement of oral reading fluency. *The original directions indicate that each word should be counted as an error. However, this practice has changed since the first publication of the Shinn (1989) text. Adapted from Shinn (1989, pp. 239–240). Copyright 1989 by The Guilford Press. Adapted by permission.

When students are reading directly from the text, bright, interesting pictures or other stimuli (e.g., brief questions about what was just read embedded within particular passages) should be eliminated, because they may disrupt continuous, fluent reading. The other disadvantage is that they may provide clues to the reader, which can undercut your ability to estimate the reader's ability to read the words (not clues) on a page. Additionally, care should be taken to avoid requiring students to read from multiple pages, because their reading rates may be reduced by this added task, especially if they do not turn pages fluently (e.g., pages stick). Passages can be shortened to the first 150 words or so and then retyped on a separate page with a reasonably sized font (e.g., 14-point Times New Roman). Be sure the probe does not exceed one page. Making an *examiner copy* with a cumulative total of words at the end of each line in the right margin makes scoring much less time consuming. *Student copies* do not have numbers in the right-hand column. You will find a sample CBM probe, including both examiner and student copies, in Figure 4.2. When you are developing materials, you also may want to use readability formulas to estimate the difficulty level of the passages. Our experience with these formulas has led us to believe that they are of limited value because they predict poorly difficulty level of passages across students. Nonetheless, you can obtain readability estimates rather simply by using the online program "Okapi" at the *interventioncentral.org* website. Just paste the passage into the Okapi program, and it reports readability.

Of the different types of probes discussed below, there are two basic categories: either the probes come from the student's curriculum or they don't. If you are looking for passages from a specific curriculum (e.g., Scott Foresman), the easiest way to prepare materials is to find someone else who already did the work. Thanks to an increasing recognition of the importance of reading fluency and its assessment, more and more publishers are preparing probes for customers. You may want to check the support materials provided with teachers' editions or contact the publisher to see if probes have already been developed. If the publisher does not have the materials, you may find other professionals nearby (e.g., special educators, school psychologists, students in local training programs in school psychology) who have already prepared materials in the curriculum you want.

With respect to choosing noncurricular materials, anything that is *not* from the student's curriculum but represents the same assessment level (e.g., fourth grade) can serve as a source of materials. This criterion makes finding materials easy. For example, if the student is using the Houghton Mifflin series, then you can use the Open Court series for

EXAMINER COPY

Some bears are brown and some are black.	8
A polar bear is white and lives by water and ice	19
and snow. A baby polar bear is born in a den.	30
The small bear stays by his mother. He likes to	40
play in the snow. He stands up on his back legs to	52
look over the ice. He calls to his mother and runs	63
over to her.	66

STUDENT COPY

Some bears are brown and some are black.
A polar bear is white and lives by water and ice
and snow. A baby polar bear is born in a den.
The small bear stays by his mother. He likes to
play in the snow. He stands up on his back legs to
look over the ice. He calls to his mother and runs
over to her.

FIGURE 4.2. Example of examiner and student copies of a CBM passage or "probe."

TABLE 4.2. Three Purposes of Oral Reading Fluency Assessments and Types and Qualities of Probes

Purposes	Sensitivity to instructional effects ← → Degree of generalization			
	Current instructional passages	High-content-overlap passages	Pool of 30 representative curricular passages	Pool of 30 independent passages of equivalent difficulty
1. Identify relative difficulty of current level (grade) of instruction.			√	
2. Gauge short-term growth.	√	√		
3. Gauge long-term growth.			√	√

noncurricular passages. Graded passages that are intended for oral reading fluency assessments can be purchased from Edformation (at *Edformation.com*), the DIBELS website (*http://dibels.uoregon.edu*, also available through Sopris West publishers), or Children's Educational Services (*http://www.readingprogress.com/*). CBM passages also can be found at *interventioncentral.org* under the "CBM Warehouse" section. Other available series are the *Timed Readings in Literature Series* (Spargo, 1989b), which include multiple-choice comprehension questions.

The selection of materials for assessment is determined by what you want to accomplish in the assessment. Here we address the selection of passages for each of the three purposes of reading fluency assessments (Table 4.2). If you want to determine a student's reading proficiency at the level at which he or she is currently being instructed, you will need a representative sample of passages from the curriculum. If you choose only passages that have been taught, you cannot really generalize the results to passages that have not yet been covered. Basically, you want to select a sample of passages from the curriculum that will give you an accurate picture of a student's skills at any point in time. This means that the results are not unduly influenced by factors that will make you overestimate or underestimate the difficulty level of the passages. There are two ways you can proceed. One strategy is to choose one passage from the beginning, one passage from the middle, and one passage from the end of the series (Shapiro, 2004). Another strategy is to generate a pool of at least 30 passages from the curriculum. If, for example, the student is reading at a second-grade level and there are two reading books at that level, you should randomly choose 30 passages from across both books, then choose three passages randomly from the total pool. Both methods help you reduce the chances of such factors as recent instruction in a particular passage significantly influencing outcomes. The advantages of the first approach are (1) greater confidence that the range of difficulty levels in the book is covered, and (2) less work. The advantage of the second method is a long-term one: If you plan on conducting long-term growth assessment using curricular materials, you can use the data generated from the initial fluency check as a part of your progress monitoring data because the basic method for selecting materials is the same. In other words, by following the latter tactic, you also have initiated the process of long-term growth assessments.

In some cases it might be helpful to get a relatively quick assessment of the effectiveness of a particular reading intervention. You can gauge short-term growth by assessing reading fluency directly in the instructional passages that are being used by the teacher. *Instructional passages* are the texts that the teacher happens to be using at the time you are doing assessments. These passages should be very sensitive to instructional effects but will provide limited information about how well the student is generalizing newly learned words to other passages. To estimate generalization of instruction effects for newly taught words, some investigators have taken to creating parallel passages that have many of the same words but are used to create a different story (Daly, Martens, Kilmer, & Massie, 1996; Daly, Hintze, & Hamler, 2000; Jones & Wickstrom, 2002). We refer to these as high-content overlap (HCO) passages because, in these studies, there has been at least an 80% rate of word overlap between instruction passages and the generalization passages on which assessment was based. These passages take a lot of work to create, especially because you have to control difficulty level of the HCO passages so that they match the corresponding instructional passages. However, they can provide a sensitive indication of whether students can read words better across passages following instruction. An example of two passages with HCO can be found in Figure 4.3. In the example, there is an 81% word overlap between the passages.

CBM Probe Taken from **Red Star, Lesson 1a**

Bob went to a farm today. He got to see five animals.	12
He saw a cat, a dog, a horse, a fish, and a pig. It was just	28
like going to the zoo. Bob got to feed the pig. The food	41
did not look good. Bob got to play with some hay and even	54
milk a cow. It was a great day. He loved to go to the	68
farm. Bob thinks he might be a farmer when he grows up. It	81
would be the best job ever. He would be able to have fun	94
all day long. It would be great.	101

Corresponding High-Content Overlap (HCO) Probe for **Red Star, Lesson 1a**

Sam went to the zoo to see the animals. First he	11
saw lions and bears. He saw the lions sleep and	21
the bears play. Next he saw the farm animals. He	31
got to feed the horse and milk the cow. The pig	42
made Sam laugh and he loved the dog. Then	51
he saw the fish swim. He had a great day at the	63
zoo. It was fun!	67

Note: Shaded words do not appear in the original passage.

Number of nonoverlapped words in the HCO passage:	13
54/67 =	**81% overlap**

FIGURE 4.3. Example of high-content-overlap passages. Reprinted by permission of Joseph C. Witt, *www.joewitt.org*.

Why might you choose curricular over noncurricular passages? Curricular passages are likely to be more sensitive to student growth over time because they are the very texts that are being taught in the classroom. However, you will be less sure of whether mastering, for example, second-grade curricular texts generalizes to other second-grade texts. By using a noncurricular reading series you can obtain independent confirmation that performance increases are being generalized by the student to untaught stories. The disadvantage of this approach is that you will probably obtain a more limited and conservative estimate of student progress over time.

The ultimate goal of instruction is to facilitate growth over time. Growth can be documented in the passages that represent the curriculum in which a student is being instructed (Shinn, 1989), or it can be documented in passages which do *not* represent the curriculum (i.e., the student has not been exposed to the passages; Fuchs & Deno, 1994). Selecting noncurricular passages can be justified on the following grounds. Ideally, an effective intervention should impact a student's reading fluency in *all* passages of equal difficulty level. If intervention effects are observed in independent passages over time (i.e., equal in difficulty level but not directly taught to the reader), you can be much more confident about the effectiveness of the intervention.

A final note about the issue of sensitivity and generalization is in order because of its bearing on how choice of materials affects decisions regarding student outcomes (see Table 4.2). When we conduct an assessment, we want to be able to make solid generalizations to other contexts. For example, when we say that a student has mastered fourth-grade reading or that he or she is ready to move on to fifth-grade reading, we are really making a theoretical claim about how well the student can read virtually any fourth-grade reading passage—a rather broad generalization. Being able to make broad generalizations comes at a price. Measurements tend to be less sensitive to recent changes in performance. Knowing that a student reads fourth-grade passages at a rate of 90 CRW per minute doesn't tell us about how well the student is responding to recent instructional efforts. To answer this question, we need a more sensitive measure. Determining that the student progressed from 75 CRW per minute to 145 CRW per minute following instruction gives us information about how well the student is responding to instruction. A more restricted generalization is being made here.

More sensitive measures have some advantages. First, if a student is *not* progressing, you can be sure that the intervention is not working, allowing you to come to a conclusion rather quickly. Second, sensitive measures tend to encourage stakeholders when a student progresses, which might help the student progress even more because others' investment in the intervention increases as a result of growth. Unfortunately, however, sensitive measures limit our ability to generalize about how the student would be performing under unassisted conditions and with other passages at different difficulty levels and possibly with different words. Herein lies the trade-off. You can't get high sensitivity and make broad generalizations at the same time, unless you measure reading fluency in different ways using different materials over time (i.e., with different explicit purposes and the different steps and procedures they entail). Of all the types of reading fluency assessments, measuring long-term growth is the most important. If you have to choose one type of assessment over others because of time or resource limitations, then long-term progress monitoring should be your highest priority.

Steps and Interpretation of Oral Reading Fluency Assessments

The steps for conducting each type of assessment and how to interpret the results are described in Table 4.3. The first task, identifying the relative difficulty of the current instructional level, may tell you whether the material being taught to the student is too hard. Judging whether materials are too hard is itself a hard task. Unfortunately, the guidelines for instructional levels in the research literature are generally based either on expert opinion or on average fluency estimates for samples of students (i.e., norms). There are at least a couple of disadvantages with this information. First, there are differences among expert opinions and with various norms. Second, and more importantly, expert opinions and norms don't really tell us what the most beneficial fluency level is for students. Some students may progress further using harder materials, whereas other students may progress further using easier materials. Relative progress is less a matter of normative rates than it is a matter of the student's skills before instruction and the strength of instruction. Therefore, we are cautious about making strong recommendations in this area.

Nonetheless, because it is important to have a perspective on expected reading fluency levels, we have pulled together data and recommendations from several reports in the literature (see Table 4.4). There are three sets of recommendations for instructional or expected fluency levels. (Howell and Nolet [2000] refer to their guidelines as expected fluency rates.) The second part of the table describes average fluency rates that have been obtained at various times in the Minneapolis school district. Specifically, the rates reported by Hasbrouck and Tindal (1992) are based on data collected on between 7,000 and 9,000 students. The actual scores are the medians for the 50th to the 75th percentiles. The rates reported by Marston and Magnusson (1988) are based on 2,720 students for each testing period (resulting in a total standardization sample of 8,160 students) in Minneapolis, Minnesota. (The numbers in parentheses are standard deviations. All numbers in the first two parts of the table were rounded to the nearest whole number.) A comparison of these figures reveals a relatively high degree of correspondence between fluency rates. Of course, they are based on students in the same geographical area. However, our experience with developing local norms and comparing these figures to others that have appeared in the literature suggests that these fluency rates are robust and give a good, general indication of the level at which the average student is reading.

For the following reasons, we suggest that you use these instructional placement recommendations and average fluency rates as guidelines *only* for what to expect. By triangulating information across sources and with increasing experience and perhaps local norms (Shinn, 1989), you will be able to judge good from poor performance. We advise against using this information as the basis of making hard-and-fast rules about student placement levels. Consider that when designing interventions, consultants tend to have little power over the level at which students are being taught. Teachers are often resistant to moving a child down in the curriculum because it would create yet more reading groups. Therefore, as a consultant, the best you may be able to do is to assist in developing an intervention at the current level at which the student is being taught. Besides, there is no guarantee that an intervention in the student's current instructional level is going to be any less effective than an intervention at a lower instructional level.

TABLE 4.3. Conducting Oral Reading Fluency Assessments: Steps and Interpretation

Purpose/task	Steps	Considerations and interpretation
1. Identify relative difficulty of current level (grade) of instruction.	• Ask the teacher for the grade or reading series level at which the student is being instructed. • Choose three probes either from the beginning, middle, and end of the book, or randomly from all appropriate passages. • Administer and score three passages. • Identify median CRW and errors per minute. • Repeat assessment and scoring if time permits and if consistency (reliability) of results is to be evaluated.	• *Grades 1–3:* If the student is reading 30 or fewer CRW per minute, then the reading material used for instruction is probably very difficult for him or her. Very strong intervention (i.e., multiple components and emphasis on acquisition) or moving down in the curriculum is wise. We recommend using Howell and Nolet's (2000) upper-bound fluency rates (e.g., 50 at grade 1, 100 at grade 2, 140 at grade 3) for setting performance goals. • *Grades 4 and above:* If the student is reading 50 or fewer CRW per minute, then the reading material used for instruction is probably very difficult for him or her. Very strong intervention (i.e., multiple components and emphasis on acquisition) or moving down in the curriculum is wise. We recommend using Howell and Nolet's (2000) upper-bound fluency rates (e.g., 100 at grade 4, 140 at grades 5 and 6) for setting performance goals.
2. Gauge short-term growth.	• Identify four to six upcoming instructional passages and create multiple probes (instructional or HCO) of each. • Establish a baseline in all probes: Administer all probes for 1 minute on two or three separate days *prior* to instruction in any of the passages. • Identify the schedule of instruction for each passage (i.e., the order of instruction and number of days each passage will be instructed).	• This method allows you to determine performance increases in response to treatment in passages over time. • If there is a visible increase in level and/or trend relative to baseline levels and trends, the intervention appears to be having immediate effects and may increase generalized performance over time. If there is not a visible increase in level or trend, strengthen the intervention (i.e., add other components) or choose another intervention.

- Establish trends once instruction has begun: Repeatedly assess reading fluency (1 minute) in (1) current passage being taught, (2) at least one as-yet-untaught passage (randomly chosen), and (3) one already-taught passage (once instruction in the first passage has been completed; randomly chosen).
- Gather at least two or three assessment data points for each passage *during* instruction while concurrently gathering pre- and postinstruction data on other passages.

3. Gauge long-term growth.

- Identify 30 equally difficult reading probes as the pool for selecting assessment materials.
- Randomly choose three probes for each assessment two times a week.
- Administer and score the three probes.
- Identify median CRW and errors per minute.
- Replace probes in the pool to be used again.

- By sequentially modifying the treatment across passages, this method can be used to compare two treatments or to examine the effects of adding or subtracting intervention components. Interpretation needs to be adjusted according to any differences in baselines across passages in which treatments are being compared.
- Immediate performance increases in no way guarantee long-term effects. However, the absence of such effects should cast doubt on the efficacy of the intervention.

- Changes in trend and level over time (or their absence) indicate whether generalized increases and maintenance are occurring.
- If the student is not making increases of three CRW per minute a week, then chances of that student "catching up" are significantly reduced. A determination of performance increases should be made after 10 data points.
- Using curricular passages is more likely to be sensitive to instructional effects (i.e., the student is being taught the passages) while still providing a reasonable estimate of generalized increases.
- Using noncurricular passages of equal difficulty level is less likely to be sensitive to instructional effects, making it a more conservative estimate of growth in oral reading fluency. However, performance increases would suggest greater efficacy of the intervention to affect untaught but equivalent passages (generalization).

TABLE 4.4. Instructional Placement Recommendations, Average Fluency Rates, and Average Words per Minute Increase per Week in Oral Reading Fluency

Study	Grade 1			Grade 2			Grade 3			Grade 4			Grade 5			Grade 6		
	Fall	Win.	Spr.	Fall	Win.	Spr.	Fall	Win.	Spr.	Fall	Win.	Spr.	Fall	Win.	Spr.	Fall	Win.	Spr.
Instructional placement recommendations																		
Fuchs & Deno (1982)	30–49 CRW 3–7 errors			30–49 CRW 3–7 errors			30–49 CRW 3–7 errors			50–99 CRW 3–7 errors			50–99 CRW 3–7 errors			50–99 CRW 3–7 errors		
Howell & Nolet (2000)	30–50 CRW < 4 errors			70–100 CRW < 6 errors			110–140 CRW < 8 errors			> 140 CRW < 8 errors			> 140 CRW < 8 errors			> 140 CRW < 8 errors		
Shapiro (2004a)	40–60 CRW < 5 errors			40–60 CRW < 5 errors			70–100 CRW < 7 errors			70–100 CRW < 7 errors			70–100 CRW < 7 errors			70–100 CRW < 7 errors		
Average fluency rates																		
Hasbrouck & Tindal (1992)				53–82	78–106	94–124	79–107	93–123	114–142	99–125	112–133	118–143	105–126	118–143	128–151			
Marston & Magnusson (1988)	19 (36)	52 (50)	71 (39)	51 (41)	73 (44)	82 (39)	88 (40)	107 (41)	115 (38)	105 (42)	115 (41)	118 (43)	118 (40)	129 (43)	134 (40)	115 (39)	120 (37)	131 (39)
Average words per minute increase per week (slope)																		
Deno et al. (2001)	1.80 (.15)			1.66 (.09)			1.18 (.10)			1.01 (.05)			0.58 (.05)			0.66 (.04)		
Fuchs et al. (1993)	2.10 (.80)			1.43 (.69)			1.08 (.52)			0.84 (.30)			0.49 (.28)			0.32 (.33)		
Marston & Tindal (1995)	2–3			2–3			1.5–2.5			1.5–2.5			1.5–2.5			1.5–2.5		

The steps for assessing short-term growth that appear in Table 4.3 outline a method for sampling current instructional passages in a systematic way that allows you to examine how much growth occurs during and following instruction. This method has proven quite useful in both our research and clinical practice and is readily adapted to school situations when someone (e.g., a special educator, a school psychologist, a paraprofessional) is available on a regular basis to do assessments. This assessment strategy follows the logic of an experimental design (the multiple-probe design; Horner & Baer, 1978).

Basically, you (1) establish baselines in all passages and (2) concurrently gather intervention data on passages in which the student is receiving instruction and baseline data on passages that are not being taught (i.e., passages in the "queue" for instruction). For assessment purposes you can use either the instructional passages or HCO passages. The former choice simplifies preparation of materials. The latter choice gives you some index of whether generalization from instruction is occurring. You continue to assess all passages even after instruction has been completed in one or more passages (i.e., the teacher has moved on to the next story). By doing so, you obtain information about whether the student is maintaining fluency gains as a result of instruction. An example appears in Figure 4.4. In this example, each graph represents a separate passage. You can see that the second intervention (delivered in the second passage and thereafter) was stronger than the first intervention. Coordination with the teacher and frequent contact with the student are critical to the success of this assessment method.

Long-term growth assessment involves choosing probes from the pool of assessment materials over time. Stories, or probes, are chosen randomly and replaced each time an assessment is done. The more frequently assessments are conducted, the more quickly you can arrive at a decision about the effectiveness of the intervention. To make a reliable decision, you must have sufficient data points. Good and Shinn (1990) found that 10 data points were adequate. By collecting data twice weekly, you get 10 data points in 5 weeks, when a decision can be made (Shinn & Hubbard, 1992). An example of a long-term growth assessment can be found in Figure 4.5. In this example, you can see that the rapid adjustment of the intervention led to an increasing trend in performance. An adjustment was made before 10 data points were collected because the short-term assessments (Figure 4.3) revealed that the first intervention would probably not be successful.

The obvious question at this point is how much growth a student should make. Table 4.4 contains estimates of growth in words per minute per week in typical samples of students from three different reports (slopes of improvement). Deno, Fuchs, Marston, and Shin (2001) obtained performance increases of about 1.80 words per minute per week for the first graders in their sample. (The numbers in parentheses are standard errors.) You will see that students tend to make greater increases in fluency in the earlier grades than in the later grades. You will also note that there are some significant discrepancies across reports, and that there are no absolutes in this area either. Deno et al. (2001) also looked at seven reading intervention studies of students with learning disabilities. All of the studies reported significant growth in reading performance. Across these studies, the average weekly CRW per minute growth rate for the second- through sixth-grade participants was 1.39 words per minute per week. These figures may prove helpful to you in gauging the progress of students who are receiving reading interventions.

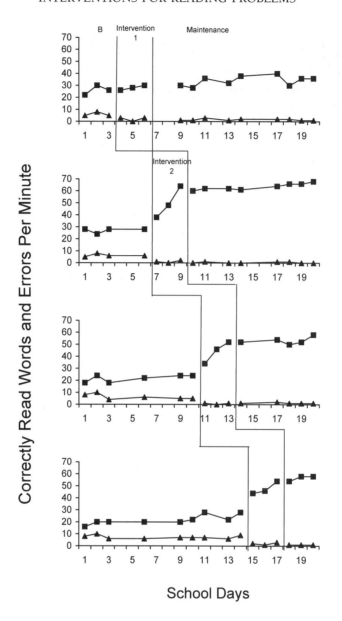

FIGURE 4.4. Example of short-term growth assessment during reading intervention.

EMPIRICALLY VALIDATED READING INTERVENTIONS

Although there may be many names for the different types of available reading interventions, they are easier to sift through when you understand that they are all variations on a small number of themes. (When someone makes a procedural change, the intervention gets a new name and is advertised as a "new and improved" strategy.) We present a manageable number of interventions that represent the fundamental principles that impact student learning. You may come across other intervention strategies in the literature, but

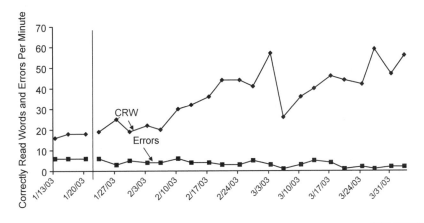

FIGURE 4.5. Example of long-term growth assessment for reading intervention.

we are confident that if you compare them to the ones presented in Table 4.5, you will see that they differ only in the degree to which they emphasize different components. One strategy might have more acquisition components, whereas another contains more fluency-building ingredients. Although we have adopted the popular names from the literature for the interventions listed in Table 4.5 and discussed briefly below, we stress their features relative to the instructional hierarchy described in Chapter 2, so that you know when an intervention is likely to be more appropriate; that is, according to whether the student is having difficulty with accuracy, fluency, or generalization.

Repeated Readings

The procedure of repeated readings is presented first because it is the intervention that will work with the largest number of students. In this procedure the student reads the same passage multiple times. The student gets a lot of practice time and the procedure is simple. Repeated reading is perhaps the purest form of the "practice makes perfect" model of enhancing reading fluency. Various studies have shown that repeated reading is an effective procedure for enhancing reading fluency in general education students as well as students with disabilities (e.g., Blum & Koskinen, 1991; Chomsky, 1978; Dowhower, 1987; Samuels, 1979; Sindelar, Monda, O'Shea, 1990). This strategy is perhaps the best fluency builder, thanks to all the practice time it affords, and can help to correct situations in which there is a lack of sufficient practice, which may be the greatest weakness of many reading curricula.

Although at first glance repeated readings may appear to produce monotony for students, our experience is that they generally like the intervention and are compliant with the procedure. One reason is that they usually get a lot of positive adult attention and encouragement for any improvement. (Be sure to praise the student for each improvement.) Students see themselves improve within passages and, because good effects are generally obtained, across passages. They see reading becoming easier and less effortful. We do, however, recommend strongly that you include a performance feedback compo-

TABLE 4.5. Overview of Basic Interventions

Type of intervention	Purpose of intervention			Appropriate uses	Limitations
	Acquisition	Fluency	Generalization		
Repeated readings		√	• To reading words in context • Potentially to other texts with the same words	• Probably the most effective intervention with the most students, because it provides many opportunities to respond.	• Does not correct errors, so students may practice errors if an error correction component is not used. • Lacks an acquisition component for reading new words. However, students who are beyond acquisition and who have decoding skills may improve on some words "spontaneously" (i.e., without explicit modeling). • May be boring for some students if there is no performance feedback and contingent positive social attention for improvements.

Procedures

1. Present a text to the student and explain that you will have him or her practice reading the passage to help him or her get better at reading.
2. Have the student read the passage aloud three or four times, or have the student read the passage aloud for a preset amount of time (e.g., 2 or 3 minutes) three or four times.

Type of intervention	Purpose of intervention			Appropriate uses	Limitations
	Acquisition	Fluency	Generalization		
Phrase drill error correction	√		• This is a very strong error correction procedure, because students practice error words in connected text. Students are more likely to generalize correct reading of words when phrase drill is used than when error correction procedures do not have students practice words in context.	• This error correction procedure addresses errors effectively and encourages students to read each and every word correctly.	• This error correction is a bit more complex procedurally than other error correction procedures, and it takes more time.

Procedures

1. Have the student read a text while you underline or highlight error words.
2. When the student has finished reading the text, show him or her your copy with the underlined/highlighted words.
3. Read the error word correctly to the student (model).
4. Have the student read the phrase/sentence containing the error word aloud three times.
5. If a sentence contains more than one error word, model correct reading of all error words in the sentence first and then have the student read the phrase/ sentence three times.

Type of intervention	Purpose of intervention			Appropriate uses	Limitations
	Acquisition	Fluency	Generalization		
Performance feedback		√	• May provide motivating conditions that help the student to want to read	• If the condition is motivating for the student, he or she takes	• Students may mistake the purpose of reading as one of just trying to read faster. It is critical to

Intervention			
	faster in the presence of the teacher/tutor, leading to generalized increases in reading when the teacher/tutor asks the student to read aloud.	an interest in trying to read faster.	stress the importance of reading words correctly and that this intervention component may help to make other reading easier, but will not, in itself, increase comprehension.

Procedures

1. Present the text to the student and explain that you will *give* feedback on how quickly and accurately he or she reads the passage.
2. Begin timing of the student when he or she says the first word. If the first word is pronounced incorrectly, correct the student and begin timing with the next word.
3. When the student has finished reading the text, give the student the following information: (a) how many words were read in the first minute, or (b) how much time it took to finish the story, and (c) how many errors he or she made.

| Listening while reading | √ | Accurate and fluent reading of connected text is modeled for the student, increasing the chances that the student will be better able to read connected text containing similar words. | • This is a strong intervention for students who have high error rates and read slowly. |

Procedures

1. Present the text to the student and tell him or her that you will read the story aloud to help the student learn how to read the words. Tell the student to follow along with his or her finger.
2. Read the text at a comfortable reading rate while monitoring the student's tracking correctly with his or her finger.
3. Have the student read the passage aloud to you.

• Students may not pay attention or practice reading subvocally while the teacher/tutor is reading the story aloud. For this reason, students generally get fewer opportunities to respond.

| Folding-in flashcard instruction | √ | • May produce generalized responding of isolated word reading, but will probably be less effective for text reading if the student does not practice newly acquired words in text through other intervention components. | • When students are not responding to interventions in connected text (i.e., error rate is high and accuracy is poor), isolating words might help them to acquire more words.
• Students get a lot of practice opportunities, and the task tends *not* to produce frustration because teaching of unknown words occurs in the context of many known words. Also, it gives the teacher/tutor ample opportunity to praise students and give positive feedback on performance. | • It is not a particularly strong strategy for producing generalized increases in reading fluency.
• The procedures require practice and may be confusing initially for teachers/consultants unfamiliar with them. |

(continued)

91

TABLE 4.5. (*continued*)

Type of intervention	Purpose of intervention			Appropriate uses	Limitations
	Acquisition	Fluency	Generalization		

Procedures

1. Identify a pool of words the student can read ("knowns") and a pool of words the student cannot read ("unknowns"). This can be done either by having a student read texts and marking error words (unknowns) and correctly read words (knowns), or by presenting words on flashcards from commonly used word lists and having the student say the words aloud, putting "corrects" and "incorrects" in separate piles.

2. Choose three unknown words for training and seven known words.

3. Modeling of unknown words: Present each of the three unknown words on flashcards and read each word to the student. Have the student read the word back to you immediately after your reading of the word. Do this for all three words.

4. When you present flashcards in the following steps, instruct the student to "say the word" (this direction can be dropped once the student understands the procedure). If the student does not say the word in 3 seconds, say the word and have the student say the word back to you. If the student responds correctly, say "Good." Present unknown and known words in the following order.

5. Present the first unknown word, followed by the first known word.

6. Present the first unknown word, followed by the first and second known words.

7. Present the first unknown word, followed by the first, second, and third known words.

8. Continue the same procedure (first unknown word, followed by knowns, until all seven knowns are presented with the first unknown), thereby "folding-in" the known words with the first unknown.

9. Repeat this process using the first two unknowns (i.e., present unknown words with known words until all seven unknown words have been presented). With respect to the order of unknown words that precedes known words, present the second unknown word first, followed by the first unknown word, followed by the first known word, etc.

10. Repeat the same process for the third unknown word, presenting the third unknown word first, the second unknown word second, and the first unknown word third, before presenting known words.

11. At the end of the session, assess student performance by (a) pooling all unknown and known words (including those that have been discarded from instruction as a result of step 12), (b) shuffling the cards, (c) presenting each card for up to 3 seconds, and (d) putting corrects (i.e., read correctly in 3 seconds) in one pile and incorrects (i.e., read incorrectly or hesitated for more than 3 seconds) in another pile. Count the number of corrects and record the score. (This step can be conducted at the beginning of subsequent sessions to test for retention across days, which might provide a more accurate estimate of what the student has learned.)

12. When a student reads a word correctly on two consecutive days during the assessment portion, make it a "known" and remove one of the previous known words to keep the number of words per session to 10. These discarded known words will still be useful in assessment (see step 11), so don't throw them away!

92

nent, such as telling a student how many words he or she read correctly in comparison to a previous reading. Students are more likely to be motivated by this kind of feedback. Because there is no acquisition component for words the student has not yet learned to read, we recommend that you include an error correction procedure, such as a phrase drill (see below) to bring the errors down across readings and reduce the risk of having students practice errors repeatedly. Finally, it is important to have students read aloud rather than silently, because students who are asked to read silently may not reread the passage (McDaniel et al., 2001; Chard, Vaughn, & Tyler, 2002). Furthermore, the students' reading performances can be measured and monitored when the reading is done orally. These data can be used to monitor progress, provide fluency feedback, and encourage students to continue reading.

Figure 4.6 shows a graph of performance feedback that can be used to enhance students' willingness to engage in repeated readings. A student's daily reading performance, wherein the student rereads the same passage three times each day, is displayed in bar graph form. The first shaded bar for each session represents the first student reading; the dark bar that follows represents the second student reading, and the white bar, the third reading for that day. The pattern of improvement shown in Figure 4.6 is fairly typical: Student performance *almost always* improves with each rereading. This improvement should be communicated to students, and they should be praised and reinforced for it.

Generalized improvement on other texts may be observed, because the student is practicing correct and rapid word reading in connected text. However, in one investigation that directly manipulated the amount of word overlap between what was taught and what was assessed, repeated readings did not produce greater increases in conditions when there was more word overlap than when there was less overlap with the same amount of practice (Rashotte & Torgesen, 1985). Yet, there have been instances reported in the litera-

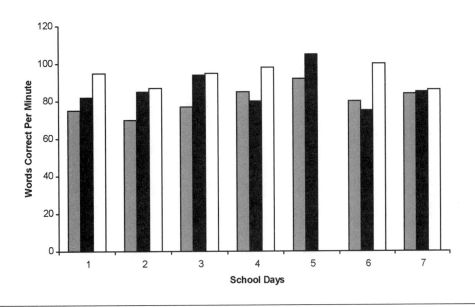

FIGURE 4.6. Example of repeated readings performance data.

ture in which generalization to noninstructed texts with high word overlap has been found with repeated readings (Daly, Martens, Dool, & Hintze, 1998; Daly & Murdoch, 2000). The bottom line is that there are no guarantees that generalized improvements will be observed. Studies that have yielded generalization increases (e.g., Daly, Martens, et al., 1996) have usually used multicomponent interventions (i.e., more than one strategy at a time). We suspect that the degree of generalization achieved with a particular student will be a function of his or her baseline skills prior to intervention and the strength of the intervention. Students whose problems are less severe and for whom attention and feedback are reinforcing are more likely to improve across passages with repeated readings.

Generalized student progress can be measured, to some degree, by assessing their reading improvement on previously unread passages. This can be done by assessing improved rates of words correct per minute during the first reading. The initial reading data (first shaded bar from each assessment) presented in the bar graphs of Figure 4.6 are presented as a line graph in Figure 4.7. These data show a less stable but increasing trend in the student's reading progress (reading rate on novel passages).

Phrase Drill Error Correction

Error words should be treated as unlearned words, even if the student can get the word right from time to time. *Unlearned words* are words that have not been acquired. In response to errors, educators generally model correct reading of the word (an acquisition strategy), prompt a response from the student (practice), and provide feedback immediately for every response (an acquisition strategy). Feedback generally comes in the form of praise for a correct response (e.g., "Correct!") or correction (e.g., "No, the word is . . . say it again"). Intervention strategies that train students in the context of connected text (as

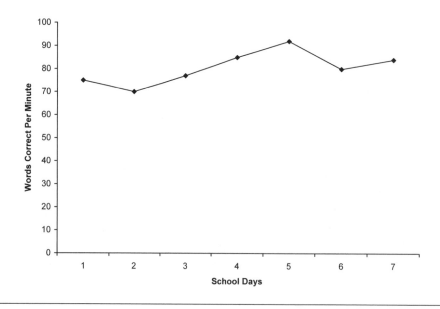

FIGURE 4.7. Example of a progress monitoring graph: Repeated readings data.

opposed to training word reading in isolation) increase the likelihood of correct reading in texts (generalization; Daly, Lentz, & Boyer, 1996; Daly & Martens, 1994). Phrase drill is superior to other error correction strategies (O'Shea, Munson, & O'Shea, 1984) for this very reason—it makes the student practice correct reading of the word in connected text (the context for reading). To use phrase drill it is necessary to have the student read an instructional passage at least once. Adding phrase drill to repeated readings makes for a very powerful intervention. When combining repeated readings and phrase drill for an individual student, we suggest that you do the phrase drill procedure after you have the student read the passage once. That way, the student practices correct reading of the words during the phrase drill procedure and also practices correct reading during the following two or three student passage readings that complete the repeated readings portion of the intervention strategy.

Performance Feedback

Performance feedback is primarily a motivational strategy that doesn't really teach students anything, except that it is important to read faster than they are currently reading. Many students like to try to beat their last score, and performance feedback might be rewarding, in itself. Using praise and encouraging statements may have even more rewarding value. If the teacher or tutor works with the student to graph his or her performance, the student can visually see increases and even gets a little math lesson as a part of the package! Results can be graphed for each reading of a passage or for the first reading and the last reading (to make it simpler; see Figure 4.6). Students are likely to see performance increases on a daily basis (i.e., from the first to last reading) and across sessions over time (as their initial reading performance increases). This tangible improvement is generally rewarding for those responsible for the intervention as well, as they get a visual representation of the student's performance over time. (There's nothing like hard data!) Performance feedback (Eckert, Ardoin, Daly, & Martens, 2002) works particularly well with repeated readings

Performance feedback can be strengthened further by the use of rewards. Performance increases can be tied to access to privileges (e.g., extra free time, being line leader, reduced work load, having lunch with the teacher, not having lunch with the teacher), tangibles (e.g., selecting an object or toy from a treasure chest, much like at the dentist's office), and social praise from significant individuals (e.g., showing the student's reading score to the principal). In one study, performance feedback and access to tangible rewards were used to influence middle school students with behavioral disorders to *choose* which type of instruction they would receive (Daly, Garbacz, Olson, Persampieri, & Ni, in press). The students had no obligation to choose to practice or do anything before they could try to go for a reward. Although reward criteria were different for students according to their skill level, the participants almost always *chose* the procedure in which experimenters had them practice, correct their errors, and model reading for them (on occasion). Performance increases in reading fluency across passages were found. In this study, performance feedback was critical to indicating to the students whether their practice was helping them and for determining whether they met their goals.

Modeling: Listening while Reading

Listening while reading (LWR) is another effective and simple procedure for enhancing oral reading. (This procedure also has been referred to as listening previewing [Rose, 1984a] and assisted reading [Hoskisson & Krohm, 1974].) During LWR, students first are instructed to read along silently as another reads aloud. The student then rereads the same passage. LWR has been shown to enhance oral reading in students who have learning disabilities in reading or mental retardation (Daly & Martens, 1994; Rose, 1984a, 1984b, 1984c). LWR has been used to enhance students' speed of accurate reading across passages and word lists (Freeman & McLaughlin, 1984; Skinner, Cooper, & Cole, 1997). The effect of LWR on fluency is probably more indirect and not as strong as those of repeated readings. The modeling component (i.e., reading to the student) is primarily an acquisition strategy, which may help the student get the words right during subsequent practice (i.e., the student-reading portion of the procedure). However, the procedure provides a limited amount of practice, and it is practice that strengthens learning more than anything else (just ask a piano teacher!).

Findings from several studies suggest that during LWR interventions, it is critical that the rate of oral presentation be slow enough so that the students who are following along have sufficient time to read silently, attempt to read, and use the model reading as accuracy feedback to the printed material (Skinner et al., 1993; Skinner, Cooper, et al., 1997; Skinner & Shapiro, 1989; also see Skinner, Logan, Robinson, & Robinson, 1997 for a review). It is best if oral readers do not read much faster than the students' current reading rate. Fluent readers who intentionally reduce their reading rates should avoid reading in a clipped, word-by-word fashion. Instead, they should read according to the rhythm of the material, pausing appropriately for punctuation marks and using inflection. The greatest problem we have found with this approach is that students may not pay full attention and therefore may derive limited benefits from the modeling. We expected the modeling to make it a strong procedure, but we have seen many students who do better with the repeated readings intervention than with the LWR intervention. Of course, the issue needs to be resolved on a case-by-case basis, and there are no strong predictors of how a student will do with the interventions, short of trying them both and seeing how he or she responds to each.

Teaching Words in Isolation: Folding-In

In general, students progress more when they practice reading connected text, the natural context in which words appear. So, as noted above, the intervention strategies that train word reading in connected text are more likely to promote generalization across texts. In some cases, however, the connected text creates too much "busyness" for a student to be able to learn individual words. Indeed, in some instances teaching in context may create more confusion (Howell & Nolet, 2000). When this is the case, it is better to teach a student to read words in isolation. Teaching words in isolation may help the student to focus on each word's properties and not get distracted by all the other words surrounding the word to be learned. This is where flashcards can be useful, because they provide opportunities for the student to practice reading words in isolation. As proficiency with words on flashcards increases, the teacher or tutor can increase the pace of presentation. Being able to read a word on a flashcard is entirely dependent on knowing the properties of the word and not on context—an important step toward making word reading more automatic.

Although there are a number of ways that flashcard instruction can be conducted, folding-in is probably the strongest method (Daly et al., 2000; MacQuarrie, Tucker, Burns, & Hartman, 2002; Shapiro, 2004a, 2004b). Folding-in involves having the student respond to both known and unknown words on flashcards; unknown words are "folded in" to the known words. Most of the words used in a teaching session are known words. Therefore, the student has a high success rate and practices already learned material while learning new material. Although the teacher or tutor spends a lot of time folding in words the student already knows, there are at least two benefits for this additional effort: First, the added practice with these known words helps the student to build fluency, and second, it makes the overall task easier than if you are presenting only unknown words. Laboriously practicing unknown words can become tedious. When there is the reinforcement of making some correct responses, students find the task to be less challenging and more rewarding—which may increase their motivation.

Flashcards are helpful, however, only if the student ultimately learns to read the words in connected text. Therefore, folding-in should probably not be used by itself, as you are not likely to see generalization to connected text without additional intervention steps. For folding-in exercises you can identify both known and unknown words based on the student's reading of story passages in curricular materials. Simply note incorrect words as the student reads a passage. Next, write down all the unknown words and seven known words. Then, you can create a folding-in passage with words from curricular material. After the student has begun to acquire unknown words, you can have him or her practice the words in connected text with the other intervention components (e.g., repeated readings, listening while reading) described above.

THE CONTEXT FOR READING INTERVENTION: PUTTING THE COMPONENTS TOGETHER

You now have some ideas and some steps to follow for creating reading interventions. The problem is figuring out which strategies are most appropriate for each student. Psychology has had a long love affair with attempting to predict successful interventions. Unfortunately, the practice went way beyond the data, and researchers and practitioners alike forgot to check the outcomes before coming up with complicated processes for prescribing interventions (Kavale & Forness, 1999). There are no sure ways to predict which strategy or combination of strategies is going to work. You simply have to choose them and try them. That's why long-term progress monitoring is the most important form of assessment. Each case is essentially a new experiment, and there will be differences in circumstances both within and across cases. What is highly effective for one child might not be effective for another child, and what works at one time with a child might not work as well at another. Therefore, we acknowledge that the best we can do is give you some guidelines that may save you time in the long run. It is your responsibility to monitor the intervention carefully and make adjustments, as necessary.

In this last section of the chapter, we (1) make general recommendations for maximizing the success of intervention sessions, (2) provide guidelines for knowing when to choose which intervention strategies, and (3) describe two different interventions in some detail (one that is appropriate for students who are struggling significantly with basic phonics skills, and one that is appropriate for classroom intervention).

The best way to improve students' reading is by making them read! You may be thinking that this is an overly obvious suggestion. However, one of the characteristics of poor classroom instruction is a lack of active student responding (i.e., student reading). Often, students who are having difficulty learning to read spend *less* rather than *more* time reading in the classroom. Intervention sessions should be characterized by *a lot* of active student responding. Students should spend most of the time reading something. Students who are not actively reading aloud during instruction should be engaging in activities that prepare them to read aloud (e.g., following a model of good reading so that the passage becomes easier to read). Such sessions should not be too long; students are likely to become fatigued and frustrated if sessions last more than about 20 minutes, in general. Of course, some students won't be able to sustain attention even that long. You will need to monitor each child carefully.

We also suggest that you attempt to integrate intervention procedures with current ongoing instruction as much as possible. For instance, repeated readings can be handled by a tutor or willing parent before or after a child reads a story in reading group. Folding-in words can be taken from reading passages, and so forth. View these intervention strategies as ways to supplement what is currently happening in the classroom. There are exceptions to this rule, however. We have seen examples where a teacher is willing to revise classroom instruction procedures altogether because he or she recognizes that more children will benefit. In this case, ongoing instruction is changed to fit the chosen intervention strategies. Perhaps, for example, the teacher is willing to do repeated readings with the reading group through a choral reading exercise (i.e., all students reading aloud together). Another situation arises when a student's skill level is significantly below the current instructional level—for example, a third-grade student receiving second-grade instruction but still showing significant deficits in phoneme segmenting abilities or phonics skills. The intervention should probably target these prerequisite skills. You may want to work with the teacher to see if he or she can modify work demands (e.g., seatwork) so that the student is working on material that is at a more appropriate level.

Another approach to strengthening instruction is to supplement the instruction delivered by the teacher with an intervention that is carried out by the student, a peer, someone at home, or another adult (e.g., a volunteer tutor or an available paraprofessional; Lentz, Allen, & Ehrhardt, 1996). If a peer or a volunteer is trained to do repeated readings, LWR, or error correction with the target student, tutoring sessions can occur *before* the student arrives in reading group, making him or her more capable of benefiting from the instruction the teacher is delivering. Alternately, the teacher can assign passages or words to be reviewed through one or more of the interventions outlined in Table 4.5 *after* instruction for practice and more in-depth error correction. Teachers need not bear all the burden of instructional interventions. Utilizing available resources wisely can help to improve the impact of the teacher's instruction.

Prioritizing Intervention Strategies

When choosing which intervention to use, you need to balance effectiveness with cost efficiency (in terms of time and resources). In many cases, a simpler intervention is a good starting point. Avoid making recommendations to a teacher for interventions that are cumbersome and difficult to manage—unless, of course, they are absolutely necessary. If a simpler intervention does not work, then try a more complex one (which might involve nothing more than adding intervention components, as opposed to changing the intervention entirely). That said, the ground rule is: Start with a simpler intervention that is likely to be effective most of the time. The intervention of repeated readings fits this requirement well. Repeated readings often is the strongest fluency-building intervention of those discussed in this chapter. The other strategies support or enhance the efficacy of repeated readings.

Where do you go from this point in the process? What else might you add? There are a few more factors you might consider in terms of prioritizing intervention components. Table 4.6 presents our recommendations for how you might prioritize the choice of additional intervention strategies. You will want to vary intervention components depending on the student's skill level. If a student is at more of an acquisition level than a fluency level, then there are additional steps you probably should take. A more significant problem occurs when a student is struggling with basic phonics and having difficulty reading even the simplest texts. The table characterizes this skill level as "phonics acquisition." An intervention plan is presented in the next section for this special case. Another factor to consider is the intensity of the intervention—that is, how much time can (and should) be put into individual reading sessions. The more intense the problem (e.g., there is a very large discrepancy with peer levels), the more intense the intervention should be. Because there are no sure predictors of intervention effectiveness, it is generally safe to start with a lower-intensity intervention and modify it if it doesn't work, rather than starting with a very intense intervention that may have some unnecessary steps. Intervention components are presented in Table 4.6 in terms of recommended levels of increasing intensity.

As you consider how much time, effort, and complexity intervention strategies are likely to add to an intervention session, you may discover that some of them really don't

TABLE 4.6. Prioritizing Intervention Components

Student's skill level	Increasing intensity ⟶				
Fluency	RR	PF	PD		
Acquisition	RR	PF	PD	LWR	F-I
Phonics acquisition	RR	PF	PD	LWR	PWI

Note. RR, repeated readings; PF, performance feedback; PD, phrase drill; LWR, listening while reading; F-I, folding-in; PWI, phonics words taught in isolation.

"cost" much. For example, performance feedback is easily added to repeated readings at very little cost in terms of time and effort—and there may be a big payoff for the student if he or she finds the improvements rewarding or if it leads to other rewards (e.g., the tutor praising the child). Although we highly recommend this strategy, a glaring weakness of it is that sometimes students end up practicing their errors. Therefore, although phrase drill is a bit more involved in terms of the time it adds to the intervention and the need for more careful supervision, it may be a worthwhile and important addition to an intervention comprised of repeated readings plus performance feedback.

If the student is really struggling or has a low fluency rate, you probably want to add some acquisition components. LWR is a relatively simple addition to an intervention plan and is easier to do than folding-in. We suggest that you add LWR first. If the student continues to have difficulty mastering some words, then start doing the folding-in procedure. You may go through some or all of these interventions and discover that the student is not responding, or you may figure out early in the process that the student hasn't mastered basic phonics skills. In that case, you might want to try something different (a recommendation is presented in the next section). Before these types of problems are addressed, we draw your attention to Worksheet 4.3, which can help you select an intervention package. You can use this form to record critical information about the case and to guide your selection of various intervention components. Figure 4.8 shows a sample worksheet that has been filled in for "Michael." In this example, Michael is presumed to have a fluency problem, and repeated readings and performance feedback are selected as interventions.

When You Can't Go Lower in the Curricular Basal Series

Figure 4.9 presents an intervention that can be used when a student is learning basic phonics skills. Although this protocol targets short-vowel sounds, it can be modified for any other type of phonic skill (e.g., long-vowel words). Just change the rule in steps 1 and 2 of Part I (the phonics lesson) to reflect the skill being taught. A variation of this intervention was used by Daly, Martens, et al. (1996) to produce generalized increases in reading fluency for HCO passages. The intervention has been changed to include a phrase drill component and performance feedback, which were not a part of the original study. The basic sequence of instruction was configured to reflect strong instructional design principles (Grossen & Carnine, 1991): The phonics skill is taught in isolation first, with opportunities to apply and practice the skill in the context of connected text. Throughout the session the student receives modeling, practice, error correction, and performance feedback. This intervention may prove particularly useful when there is no systematic teaching of phonics in the classroom.

Classwide Peer Tutoring

Repeated readings and LWR are effective procedures for enhancing reading fluency. These procedures are likely to be more effective when (1) students are reading from material that is not too difficult, (2) feedback and reinforcement are provided for improved performance, and (3) procedures are implemented frequently so that students have many

Selecting an Intervention Package

Student Name: _Michael_   Date: _1/30_

Grade: _3rd_

Step 1. Identify student needs.

Baseline student data:

Two assessments in fourth-grade basal reader; median CRW = 50, errors = 3 (1/25/04);

median CRW = 46, errors = 5 (1/27/04). Teacher notes Michael often appears unmotivated

to read.

Suggest that student is struggling with:

(Fluency)   Acquisition   Phonics Acquisition

Step 2. Select intervention strategies.

What is the simplest yet potentially appropriate package to begin with?

Skill level	Increasing intensity ⟶				
Fluency	(RR)	(PF)	(PD)		
Acquisition	RR	PF	PD	LWR	F-I
Phonics acquisition	RR	PF	PD	LWR	PWI

RR, repeated readings; PF, performance feedback; PD, phrase drill; LWR, listening while reading; F-I, folding-in; PWI, phonics words taught in isolation.

Michael needs practice and may increase motivation with performance feedback. Error rate is high

and needs to be reduced.

Step 3. General considerations.

How can the selected intervention procedures fit with current instruction, or vice versa?

Mom has agreed to supervise him at night and conduct PD after first reading. Michael and Mom

will graph the results together. They will practice upcoming stories in the curriculum. That way,

he will come to reading group well prepared.

When will the intervention be carried out and for how long each time? (Student should be reading actively during most of the session. Sessions should probably last no longer than 20 minutes.)

Michael and Mom will practice four nights a week for about 15 minutes.

FIGURE 4.8. Example of a completed worksheet for selecting an intervention package for Michael.

Overview:

1. Teach a phonics lesson.
2. Train phonics words in isolation: model plus prompt responses.
3. Have students practice phonics words in passage: model, repeated readings, error correction, performance feedback.

Materials Needed:

Instructions for administration
Instructional word list
Phonics passage
Stopwatch
Pen or pencil

Procedures:

Part I: Phonics Lesson

1. Say, "TODAY WE ARE GOING TO LEARN WORDS THAT CONTAIN THE [STATE LETTER SOUND] SOUND."

2. Present the word list to the student and say, "THESE WORDS ALL CONTAIN THE [STATE LETTER SOUND] SOUND BECAUSE . . . THE VOWEL STANDS BY ITSELF IN THE WORD AND IS SHORT."

3. Say, "I WILL READ THE WORDS TO YOU. I WANT YOU TO POINT TO THE WORDS AS I SAY THEM AND SAY THEM TO YOURSELF."

4. Read the words out loud to the student, as the student points to the words.

5. After reading the list to the student, say, "NOW I WANT YOU TO READ THE WORDS TO ME. IF YOU ARE NOT SURE OF A WORD, I WILL HELP YOU."

6. Tell the student to begin reading at the top of the list.

7. If the student does not read a word within 3 seconds, say the word for the student and have the student repeat the word (saying "Repeat after me!" if the student does not repeat the word spontaneously).

8. Have the student read the entire list, while you correct errors each time they occur.

Part II: Listening while Reading

1. Present the instructional passage to the student, saying, "THIS IS A STORY WITH A LOT OF WORDS THAT HAVE THE [STATE LETTER SOUND] SOUND. I WILL READ THE STORY TO YOU. PLEASE FOLLOW ALONG WITH YOUR FINGER, READING THE WORDS TO YOURSELF AS I SAY THEM. THE STORY IS CALLED. . . ."

2. Read the entire story at a comfortable reading rate, being sure that the student is following along with his or her finger.

Part III: Student Reading, with Error Correction and Performance Feedback Provided

1. Have the student reread the passage, saying, "NOW IT'S YOUR TURN TO READ THE PASSAGE. PLEASE BEGIN READING HERE [POINT TO THE BEGINNING] AND TRY TO READ EACH WORD. IF YOU COME TO A WORD YOU DON'T KNOW, I'LL TELL IT TO YOU. WHEN YOU ARE DONE, I WILL TELL YOU HOW QUICKLY AND ACCURATELY YOU READ THE PASSAGE."

2. Begin timing the student when he or she says the first word. If the first word is pronounced incorrectly, correct the student and begin timing with the next word. Underline or highlight error words as the student reads aloud.

3. If the student hesitates for more than 3 seconds, point to the word in the student's copy of the story, say the word, and underline the word.

4. When the student has finished reading the text, tell him or her either (a) how many words he or she read in the first minute or (b) how much time it took to finish the story and (c) how many errors he or she made.

5. Next, show the student your copy of the passage, with its underlined/highlighted words. Read each error word correctly to the student (modeling). Have the student read the phrase/sentence containing the error word aloud three times. [If a sentence contains more than one error word, model correct reading of all error words first and then have the student read the phrase/sentence three times.]

6. Have the student read the passage two more times. (That is, repeat steps 2 and 3 two more times. Omit underlining of error words.)

FIGURE 4.9. An intervention plan for students with poor accuracy and poor phonics skills (short-vowel words).

opportunities to respond. One program that incorporates all of these components is classwide peer tutoring (CWPT). CWPT is a group intervention that can increase the skills of many students at one time and is therefore an efficient intervention, if it is acceptable to the teacher.

CWPT programs have been developed for reading, mathematics, spelling, and content areas (Greenwood, Delquadri, & Carta, 1997). These programs are designed to enhance student skill development by eliciting high rates of active academic responding in all students within a classroom setting (Greenwood, Delquadri, & Hall, 1984). The program uses peers to supervise and provide feedback for responding, a game-like format in which rates of accurate oral reading are reinforced, and weekly progress evaluations that can be used to make educational decisions for individual students.

CWPT has been shown to increase academic engaged time and reading fluency in both general education students and students with disabilities (Kamps, Barbetta, Leonard, & Delquadri, 1994; Otis-Wilborn, 1984). The program is also associated with lower dropout rates, increases in performance on standardized achievement test scores, and reduced special education placement rates (Greenwood, 1991a, 1991b; Greenwood, Delquadri, & Hall, 1989; Harper, Maheady, Mallette, & Karnes, 1999). A protocol for CWPT is presented in Table 4.7. Further information about implementing CWPT can be obtained at *interventioncentral.org* (also see Chapter 2).

The CWPT program has several advantages over more traditional oral reading programs. In a class containing 15 students, a teacher may call students to a specific area of the room, have them sit in a circle, and take turns reading aloud (small-group round-robin reading). With all the time required for transition, students may be reading aloud and receiving feedback, reinforcement, and error correction for only 1 minute (often less). However, by using peers to provide this feedback, students can engage in such behavior for 10–15 minutes in the same time period.

TABLE 4.7. Classwide Peer-Tutoring Procedures

1. Use CBM data to determine students' highest instructional level.
2. Divide class into two teams each week.
3. Within each team assign students to dyads based on CBM results; students in each dyad should be reading from the same material.
4. Each student takes a turn reading aloud to team members for a fixed amount of time (10–15 minutes). As one student reads aloud (tutee), the other student (tutor) follows along, awarding points for correctly read sentences and immediately correcting errors (e.g., skipped line, mispronunciation).
5. If a student finishes the selected passage before the allotted time expires, he or she begins to reread the passage.
6. As students are reading, the teacher moves around the room giving bonus points for implementing procedures accurately and reading words that students are unable to decode.
7. After time is up, students switch roles and repeat the procedure.
8. Points are totaled.
9. Individual student points and team points are publicly posted; winning teams are announced each day, often followed by a round of applause.
10. This procedure is typically implemented 4 days per week; on the 5th day progress data are collected by having students read aloud for 1 minute (CBM procedures).

A second component to this program is that rewards, in the form of points, are delivered contingent upon rate of accurate responding. Additionally, in the game-type format, an unknown number of points is needed to win the game each day, and the mystery is highly motivating. All students are encouraged to do their best, of course. Fluent readers can help their team win by reading even more rapidly and accurately. Those with reading skill deficits also can contribute to their team's success by doing their best, which may make the activity more rewarding for them. Team compositions are changed frequently. Thus all students have an opportunity to be on a winning team.

The program incorporates both repeated reading and listening while reading. Additionally, although dyads read and reread the same material, it can be varied across groups of students with regard to difficulty and length. Length is of particular interest. For slower readers, passage length can be reduced so that while the tutee reads aloud, he or she has the opportunity to reread the material several times. This strategy should boost these students' total points and may improve their reading skills. Furthermore, CWPT provides an excellent format for LWR because students reading at the same instructional level read the material silently while serving as tutors.

When first implemented, CWPT is likely to require additional time as students learn the system. Additionally, classrooms are likely to get noisier, and some students may cheat (inflate points) or argue among each other. However, teachers who implement this program consistently find that they are able to adapt to the noise level and address these other concerns.

A final issue concerns the public posting of students' performances. Posting the low points of dysfluent readers is not recommended because it may encourage peers to compare their individual performances (i.e., points earned). Such comparisons are unlikely to be favorable to dysfluent readers. Instead, educators should post each team's performance. If individual student performance data are posted or announced, the data should include improvement rates, as opposed to raw scores, because dysfluent readers may actually show greater increases in performance than fluent readers.

CONCLUSIONS

This chapter gives an overview of the importance of, measurement of, and interventions for oral reading fluency. The intervention and measurement strategies are presented with guidelines for use, when appropriate. It is essential, however, that you adapt these methods to your local needs. Students have different fluency levels before intervention, and schools have different priorities and ways of organizing intervention efforts. The ultimate test of the utility of these interventions is whether they produce measurable increases in performance. With ongoing assessment, you will be able to determine whether the methods you are employing are meeting that standard. When the data suggest that something is not working, procedures should be revised until an effective plan is developed. It is worth repeating here that long-term monitoring of progress is the best test of the effectiveness of any intervention plan.

Students with reading skill deficits may approach all reading activities cautiously because of their history of failure. When working with these students, it is helpful to approach all activities with an upbeat attitude. Do not dwell on or punish errors or mistakes. Instead, attempt to keep scheduled activities moving along rapidly. When the student's performance improves, *do* provide feedback along with praise. Remember, students who associate reading activities with success and other positive experiences may be more likely to choose to read, as opposed to avoiding reading activities. The more frequently students choose to read, the greater their fluency is likely to become. As students become more fluent readers, they are more likely to choose to read in the future. This upward spiral is the goal of all procedures designed to enhance fluency.

WORKSHEET 4.1. Student Record Form: Curriculum-Based Measurement of Oral Reading Fluency

Student Name: _____ Grade/Classroom: _____

Reading Skill Level: _____ Best Time(s) for CBM Monitoring: _____

Step 1: Conduct a Survey-Level Assessment: Use this section to record the student's reading rates in progressively more difficult material.

Date:_____ Book/Reading Level: _____
	TRW	E	CRW	%CRW
A.	_____	_____	_____	_____
B.	_____	_____	_____	_____
C.	_____	_____	_____	_____

Date:_____ Book/Reading Level: _____
	TRW	E	CRW	%CRW
A.	_____	_____	_____	_____
B.	_____	_____	_____	_____
C.	_____	_____	_____	_____

Date:_____ Book/Reading Level: _____
	TRW	E	CRW	%CRW
A.	_____	_____	_____	_____
B.	_____	_____	_____	_____
C.	_____	_____	_____	_____

Date:_____ Book/Reading Level: _____
	TRW	E	CRW	%CRW
A.	_____	_____	_____	_____
B.	_____	_____	_____	_____
C.	_____	_____	_____	_____

Date:_____ Book/Reading Level: _____
	TRW	E	CRW	%CRW
A.	_____	_____	_____	_____
B.	_____	_____	_____	_____
C.	_____	_____	_____	_____

Date:_____ Book/Reading Level: _____
	TRW	E	CRW	%CRW
A.	_____	_____	_____	_____
B.	_____	_____	_____	_____
C.	_____	_____	_____	_____

Date:_____ Book/Reading Level: _____
	TRW	E	CRW	%CRW
A.	_____	_____	_____	_____
B.	_____	_____	_____	_____
C.	_____	_____	_____	_____

Table 1: Sample Estimates of 'Typical' CBM Instructional Reading Levels By Grade

Grade	Shapiro (1996) CRW Per Min	Shapiro (1996) Reading Errors	Milwaukee Public Schools (Winter 2000-2001 Local Norms) CRW Per Min for Students in 25th-75th Percentile
1......	40-60	Fewer than 5	22-64
2......	40-60	Fewer than 5	36-78
3......	70-100	Fewer than 7	47-88
4......	70-100	Fewer than 7	60-104
5......	70-100	Fewer than 7	77-121
6......	70-100	Fewer than 7	95-146

Step 2: Compute a Student Reading Goal

1. At what grade or book level will the student be monitored? (Refer to results of Step 1: *Survey-Level Assessment*)

   _____

2. What is the student's *baseline* reading rate (# correctly read words per min)? _____CRW Per Min

3. When is the *start date* to begin monitoring the student in reading? _____ / _____ / _____

4. When is the *end date* to stop monitoring the student in reading? _____ / _____ / _____

5. How many instructional weeks are there between the start and end dates? (Round to the nearest week if necessary):

   _____ Instructional Weeks

6. What do you *predict* will be the student's average increase in correctly read words per minute will be for each instructional week of the monitoring period? (See Table 2):

   _____ Weekly Increase in CRW Per Min

7. What will the student's predicted CRW *gain* in reading fluency be at the end of monitoring? (Multiply Item 5 by Item 6): _____

8. What will the student's predicted *reading rate* be at the end of the monitoring period? (Add Items 2 & 7): _____ CRW Per Min

References

Fuchs, L.S., Fuchs, D., Hamlett, C.L., Walz, L., & Germann, G. (1993). Formative evaluation of academic progress: How much growth can we expect? *School Psychology Review, 22*, 27-48.

Shapiro, E.S. (1996). *Academic skills problems: Direct assessment and intervention*. New York: Guilford Press.

(continued)

Step 3: Collect Baseline Data: Give 3 CBM reading assessments within a one-week period using monitoring-level probes.

Baseline 1

Date:_____ Book/Reading Level: _____

	TRW	E	CRW	%CRW
A.				
B.				
C.				

Baseline 2

Date:_____ Book/Reading Level: _____

	TRW	E	CRW	%CRW
A.				
B.				
C.				

Baseline 3

Date:_____ Book/Reading Level: _____

	TRW	E	CRW	%CRW
A.				
B.				
C.				

Step 4: Compete CBM Progress-Monitoring Weekly or More Frequently: Record the results of regular monitoring of the student's progress in reading fluency.

1. Date:_____ Book/Reading Level: _____

	TRW	E	CRW	%CRW
A.				
B.				
C.				

2. Date:_____ Book/Reading Level: _____

	TRW	E	CRW	%CRW
A.				
B.				
C.				

3. Date:_____ Book/Reading Level: _____

	TRW	E	CRW	%CRW
A.				
B.				
C.				

4. Date:_____ Book/Reading Level: _____

	TRW	E	CRW	%CRW
A.				
B.				
C.				

5. Date:_____ Book/Reading Level: _____

	TRW	E	CRW	%CRW
A.				
B.				
C.				

6. Date:_____ Book/Reading Level: _____

	TRW	E	CRW	%CRW
A.				
B.				
C.				

7. Date:_____ Book/Reading Level: _____

	TRW	E	CRW	%CRW
A.				
B.				
C.				

8. Date:_____ Book/Reading Level: _____

	TRW	E	CRW	%CRW
A.				
B.				
C.				

9. Date:_____ Book/Reading Level: _____

	TRW	E	CRW	%CRW
A.				
B.				
C.				

10. Date:_____ Book/Reading Level: _____

	TRW	E	CRW	%CRW
A.				
B.				
C.				

11. Date:_____ Book/Reading Level: _____

	TRW	E	CRW	%CRW
A.				
B.				
C.				

12. Date:_____ Book/Reading Level: _____

	TRW	E	CRW	%CRW
A.				
B.				
C.				

Table 2: Predictions for Rates of Reading Growth by Grade
(Fuchs, Fuchs, Hamlett, Walz, & Germann, 1993)
Increase in Correctly Read Words per Minute for Each Instructional Week

Grade Level	Realistic Weekly Goal	Ambitious Weekly Goal
Grade 1	2.0	3.0
Grade 2	1.5	2.0
Grade 3	1.0	1.5
Grade 4	0.85	1.1
Grade 5	0.5	0.8
Grade 6	0.3	0.65

WORKSHEET 4.2. Checklist for Creating CBM Probes for Reading Fluency

Does the reading passage contain . . .	Yes	No
☐ Continuous paragraphs rather than lots of dialogue or material such as poems?	_____	_____
☐ A majority of common words (as opposed to foreign or unusual words)?	_____	_____
☐ Approximately 150 words that can be typed on a single page?	_____	_____
☐ No stimuli (e.g., pictures) that may distract or provide clues to the student?	_____	_____

If you answered yes to all these questions, then this passage may be a good choice.
Proceed with making an examiner (cumulative word total down right margin) and student (no numbers) copy. Consider calculating a readability estimate for the passage by pasting an electronically formatted copy of the passage into the "Okapi" feature at *http://www.interventioncentral.org/.*

WORKSHEET 4.3. Selecting an Intervention Package

Student Name: _____   Date: _____

Grade: _____

Step 1. Identify student needs.

Baseline student data:

_____

_____

_____

_____

_____

Suggest that student is struggling with:

Fluency   Acquisition   Phonics Acquisition

Step 2. Select intervention strategies.

What is the simplest yet potentially appropriate package to begin with?

Skill level	Increasing intensity ⟶				
Fluency	RR	PF	PD		
Acquisition	RR	PF	PD	LWR	F-I
Phonics acquisition	RR	PF	PD	LWR	PWI

RR, repeated readings; PF, performance feedback; PD, phrase drill; LWR, listening while reading; F-I, folding-in; PWI, phonics words taught in isolation.

_____

_____

_____

Step 3. General considerations.

How can the selected intervention procedures fit with current instruction, or vice versa?

_____

_____

_____

_____

_____

(continued)

When will the intervention be carried out and for how long each time? (Student should be reading actively during most of the session. Sessions should probably last no longer than 20 minutes.)

_____

_____

_____

_____

5

Reading Comprehension

In earlier chapters we focused on developing prereading skills and fluent reading. Although being able to read fluently may be an important prerequisite skill, by itself it is merely a means to an end. Rather, the primary reason we read is for comprehension. Many students who develop fluent reading skills may not need additional interventions designed to enhance comprehension; for others, however, explicit procedures may be needed (Fuchs, Fuchs, Hosp, & Jenkins, 2001). Strategies for improving comprehension can be implemented before, during, or after reading. This chapter reviews a number of strategies that can be adopted to promote reading comprehension. The strategies (listed in Table 5.1) are organized according to when they can be used: prereading, during reading, or postreading (i.e., when the student has finished reading). Some strategies combine prereading, during-reading, and/or postreading procedures. Finally, assessment of comprehension is discussed.

PREREADING/PREVIEWING COMPREHENSION ACTIVITIES

A variety of prereading or previewing procedures may be implemented to clarify the purpose for reading and enhance comprehension. Prereading activities may enhance comprehension by helping students access prior knowledge related to the material. Students may read to confirm, support, accentuate, or disconfirm what they already know about the subject. Prereading procedures can help students to generate questions or hypotheses about the topic, and reading and comprehension can then be used to resolve them. Prereading activities also can be used to enhance the speed and accuracy of student reading, thereby reducing the time and effort required (Rousseau & Yung Tam, 1991). Finally, previewing activities may heighten students' interest in material and further encourage them to read.

TABLE 5.1. Reading Comprehension Strategies

When to use the strategy	Strategies
Prereading	Clarify the purpose of reading.
	Help the student to estimate the general content of the text by noting title, date of publication, author, and scanning the text.
	TELLS (Title–Examine–Look–Look–Setting strategy.
	Preteach vocabulary.
	Preteach concepts through semantic maps or story grammar.
	Carefully choose reading material and allow student choice of reading material (with some restrictions).
During reading	Promote frequent and sustained reading.
	Consider story grammar for fictional text.
	Use outlines and study guides for expository text.
	Apply strategic note taking for expository text.
	Use time lines and flowcharts for expository text.
	Make conflict charts.
	Use visualization for fictional text.
Postreading	Use summarization for both types of text.
	Use question-and-answer relationship training.
Combined strategies (prereading, during reading, and/or postreading)	Strategic note taking
	SQ3R
	Multipass
	POSSE
	Using rewards

Clarify the Purpose of Reading

Prior to reading, students are generally doing something else. Someone or something cues them to start reading. Sometimes these cues are subtle, and students are not aware of the purpose for their reading. For example, a bored student waiting in line at the water fountain might glance at a bulletin board and read a menu of lunches from 3 weeks ago. In this instance, the reason the student began reading is difficult to discern, and the goal of reading is unclear.

Prior to reading specific material, students should have an understanding of their purpose (Duke & Pearson, 2002). A child might read, for example, the sports section of the newspaper to find out whether his or her favorite team won; a history passage to increase the probability of passing an exam; or directions so that he or she can assemble a new toy. Students may read stories, comic books, or magazines for pleasure or enjoyment; to avert boredom and pass the time; to participate in discussions with parents, peers, or others about the material; or to achieve a specific goal (e.g., reading all of Shakespeare's plays).

When educators assign reading materials, they are likely to increase the probability of students choosing to read if they clarify the purpose or function of the assignment. In almost all instances, comprehension is part of the purpose. However, although clarifying the purpose of reading may increase the likelihood that students will choose to read, *comprehending* what is read is what is usually needed to sustain the reading.

Help Students Estimate the General Content of the Text

Read Title, Date of Publication, and Author

Students can be taught several ways to estimate the general content of the text. Reading the title of a text may allow students to access their prior knowledge about upcoming content. Although the title can provide clues regarding content, other prereading activities may be needed to help students form hypotheses about the content. For example, checking the date of publication may help students understand the author and historical context in which the text was written. Likewise, identifying the author and providing information about him or her may offer additional cues regarding content (Miller, 1982).

Scan the Text

Next, have students flip through the text to gain an overview of the content and nature of the text. Sections, subheadings, and subtitles contain helpful categorical information about the content. Illustrations, figures, tables, or graphs also give clues about the scope and sequence of the material (Idol-Maestas, 1985). Scanning the text to determine the total length or the length of each section allows students to set goals when reading requires multiple sessions. For example, students might scan a science text assigned as homework and determine that they will read and take notes on one section before dinner. These intermittent goals can help maintain a student's engagement with reading (Chan, Cole, & Barfett, 1987).

Scanning the text also can be used to identify important or unknown words. For example, many content area texts (e.g., biology) make this process easier by highlighting (e.g., printing in bold letters on first appearance) words, phrases, or terms that students are unlikely to know. However, even when these additional cues are not provided, students can be taught to scan the text and identify words that appear to be important or unknown (Idol-Maestas, 1985). Yet another use of scanning is to answer questions regarding the general nature of the text. For example, students can scan to determine if the material is factual or fictional. Because different kinds of texts are read differently, knowing whether the material is factual or fictional will probably influence the student's reading. When reading fiction, the focus is usually on characters and settings, and the reader probably does not know anything about the characters. When reading factual expository text, in contrast, the focus is usually on text structure and involves creating and revising summaries while reading (Duke & Pearson, 2002); here the student's prior knowledge may be used to assist with comprehension.

Teach the TELLS Procedure: Title–Examine–Look–Look–Setting

TELLS is an acronym for a previewing procedure designed to enhance comprehension of stories (Idol-Maestas, 1985). Table 5.2 provides an overview of the steps for using the TELLS procedure. A blank, reproducible form that can be used with students appears in Worksheet 5.1 (all worksheets are at the end of the chapter). Although the TELLS procedure can be used with individual students, it may actually be best to train students to use it in a group format.

The first step in the TELLS procedure is to teach students to form clues as to what the story is about by reading the *title*. A teacher may introduce the reading material by announcing the title and asking students what they think the story is about and why they think this. During this instruction, it is critical that teachers avoid giving evaluative feedback. What is critical is for students to learn that *they can form hypotheses about content by merely reading the title*. This first step is intended to encourage students to read in order to confirm or disconfirm their hypotheses.

The second step is to *examine*. Here students are taught to look at each page of the material, skimming for clues. These clues, which include illustrations, sections or subtitles, and figures or graphs, may cause readers to develop more complex hypotheses regarding the content. Other clues include the structure and layout of the text. For example, text with many quotation marks and a hand-drawn color picture of a dragon may suggest a fictional story, whereas text with many headings, subheadings, figures, and a black-and-white photograph of a living lizard may suggest that the material is factual.

During the third stage, *look*, students are taught to scan for important words. In this step, students can be taught to look for clues signaling important words, such as bold or italic font. Illustrations and captions also may help students identify important words. When an illustration depicts a particular event, students should look for important words surrounding that event. Students should be taught to look for words that are used frequently, because frequency may be a clue that these are important words to know and understand while reading the material.

During the fourth stage, students are taught to *look* for hard words—to skim, page by page, through a text looking for words they don't readily recognize. Sometimes a student

TABLE 5.2. Steps for the TELLS Previewing Procedure

• T Title	What is the title of this story? Does it give a clue as to what the story is about? What do you think it is about?
• E Examine	Look at each page of the story to find clues about the story. What did you find?
• L Look	Look for and write down important words, such as ones that are bold or used frequently. What do they mean?
• L Look	Look again through the story for hard words—words you do not know. Write them down. What do they mean?
• S Setting	Write down clues about the setting, such as the place, date, and time period. (Hint: These clues are often found in the beginning of the story.)
FACT or FICTION?	Is this a true story (fact)? Or is this a pretend story (fiction)?

may not recognize or know the meaning of a printed word but may recognize it once he or she hears it pronounced or uses decoding skills to pronounce it. In other instances, a student may not know the meaning of a word, even though he or she can accurately read it.

In the fifth stage, students are taught to skim for clues about the *setting* of the story, such as indications of places (e.g., city names), area descriptions (e.g., a park in the heart of downtown), dates, or references to time periods (e.g., "a few weeks before Christmas" or "before the invention of electricity"). Students should be instructed to focus their attention on the beginning of the story, because most settings are described early in the text.

After all the steps have been completed, the student answers one question regarding the general nature of the story. From the clues gathered during the TELLS exercise, the student should be able to predict whether the text is a true story (fact) or a pretend story (fiction).

Preteach Vocabulary

Understanding the meaning of important words would appear to be a prerequisite for comprehension. However, results are mixed on this issue. For example, Pany, Jenkins, and Schreck (1982) found that preteaching vocabulary words enhanced comprehension of single sentences using the pretaught words but had no effect on comprehension of longer text (i.e., two or three sentences). Other researchers have found that preteaching vocabulary enhances comprehension (Gaskins, Ehri, & Cress, 1996; Koltun & Biemiller, 1999), but not as much as other procedures (Bos, Anders, Filip, & Jaffe, 1989; Bos & Anders, 1990).

The first step in preteaching vocabulary is to identify which words to teach. Many reading curricula and content area texts (e.g., science texts) provide lists of vocabulary words that can be taught prior to reading a particular section. Additionally, educators can scan material to identify key words—that is, those words that are important in understanding the phrase or passage (Rousseau & Yung Tam, 1991). Finally, students can be asked to scan material and identify unknown words that appear to be important (Idol-Maestas, 1985).

Intermediate grade teachers tend to use many different procedures for teaching vocabulary (Lloyd, 1995–1996). The most common procedure is also one of the most time-efficient procedures: pronouncing the word for the student. If students have strong phonics skills, they can be asked to attempt to read unknown words aloud. In some cases, students may need to be prompted to sound out words. When time permits, teachers may encourage students to apply their decoding skills to the unknown words; they also may reteach or reinforce the use of these skills.

In many instances, hearing the word read correctly or reading the word accurately may allow students to comprehend the meaning. However, in other instances, students can accurately read a word but do not know what it means. In these situations, other procedures such as (1) providing a definition, (2) having a student look up the word in a dictionary, or (3) giving a synonym or antonym can enhance vocabulary. The teacher may use the word in a sentence or ask a student to do so. Alternately, the teacher may have students read a brief section of text containing that word and attempt to use context cues to discern the meaning of the word.

There are some potential problems with preteaching vocabulary. Students may forget the definition of words as they are reading. Because students with reading skill deficits often read more slowly, they are likely to have to maintain this information for a longer period of time, as they will not arrive at new words as quickly as others. Further complicating matters is that students with reading deficits may have difficulty remembering or recalling newly acquired information as they read (LaBerge & Samuels, 1974; Lesgold & Perfetti, 1978; Lesgold & Resnick, 1982; Wong, 1986).

There are several solutions to these problems. After students have initially learned the meaning of a word, context cues may help them recall it. Providing students with a list of these words and brief definitions or synonyms can be used to aid comprehension. A form like the one that appears in Worksheet 5.2 can be used for preteaching unknown words. Finally, providing sufficient opportunities to practice using new vocabulary words prior to asking students to read text containing these words can enhance the probability of the students remembering definitions as they read (Gravois & Gickling, 2002).

Another procedure that educators often use is to provide students with a dictionary and encourage them to look up unknown words that they come across while they are reading. Although this method is popular, it has several limitations. First, having students look up words in a dictionary has not been shown to be very effective (Bos et al., 1989). In many instances, it disrupts reading and interferes with comprehension, as the effort and time required to look up words causes their understanding of previously read material to deteriorate (Stanovich, 1986).

Looking up words in a dictionary also reduces time available for students to read and build their comprehension skills. Requiring students to look up words makes reading more effortful and can decrease their motivation to read. Therefore, when students are reading for comprehension, it is appropriate for educators, parents, peers, siblings, or others to provide synonyms or brief definitions of words rather than requiring the reader to look them up in the dictionary.

In some instances, students may use word analysis skills to determine meanings of words; for example, by understanding prefixes, suffixes, and root words. Providing students with grammar-related information about words (e.g., parts of speech) may assist with comprehension. Again, this should be done prior to reading for comprehension, because teaching these activities will disrupt their continuous reading and adversely affect comprehension.

Preteach Concepts

Teaching new words in isolation can be effective, as noted, but prereading procedures that teach more detailed concepts and multiple words or phases may lead to even greater increases in comprehension (Bos et al., 1989). Graphic aids or advanced organizers and semantic maps of information that is contained in the text may help students learn concepts and understand written text. These are typically graphic representations. These materials can provide students with information that enhances comprehension levels and reduces the time and effort required to comprehend. They may also help students to draw upon prior knowledge and highlight purposes for reading the text.

Before discussing the procedures for preteaching concepts, it is important to note that these materials should *supplement* but not replace the text. If advanced organizers contain all the pertinent information in the text, then there is no reason to read the text in the first place. All students, especially students with poor reading skills who require more time and must marshal more effort to read, may be more likely to choose to *not* read the text if merely studying the advanced organizer would suffice.

Semantic Maps

Semantic maps and semantic analysis charts are the most common types of graphic organizers. They can be used prior to or during reading exercises. In order to use these graphic organizers as a prereading activity, educators must create either a semantic map or semantic analysis chart. Both of these graphic organizers help to display relationships between concepts in the form of a "relationship chart." The steps used by Bos and colleagues (1989) to create these charts are summarized in Table 5.3.

The first step in developing a relationship chart is to read the assigned material and complete a content analysis. The content analysis consists of several steps during which special attention is given to textual cues (e.g., titles, subheadings, highlighted words, figures). First, the teacher must list the key concepts and vocabulary. This list is then evaluated to determine which idea seems to be all-inclusive. The *all-inclusive* topic is considered the superordinate concept (i.e., topic of the chapter) and is used as the title of the graphic organizer. The remaining entries on the list are then organized into categories. For example, the concepts can be organized into categories of characteristics, functions, examples of the main concept, or steps in a process. The main concepts for each category become the *coordinate concepts*. The remaining concepts are considered the *subordinate*,

---

TABLE 5.3. Steps in Constructing Semantic Graphs

1. Read assigned text.
2. List key concepts and vocabulary.
3. Review concept list for the all-inclusive idea (e.g., chapter topic).
4. The all-inclusive idea becomes the title of the semantic graph.
5. Organize entries on the concept and vocabulary list into categories (e.g., characteristics, steps in a process, examples of the main concept, functions).
6. The main concept for each category becomes a coordinate concept.
7. Place the coordinate concepts along the top line of the semantic graph or in the medium-sized circles of a semantic map.
8. The supporting concepts and vocabulary for each coordinate category become the subordinate concepts.
9. Place subordinate concepts along the left-hand column of the graph or in the small-sized circles underneath the coordinate circles in the semantic map.
10. Fill in the relationships between the coordinate concepts and the subordinate concepts on the graph, or fill in the relationship lines between the coordinate concepts and the subordinate concepts on the semantic map.

Note. Data from Bos, Adners, Filip, and Jaffe (1989).

or supporting *concepts* of the coordinate concepts. Those concepts that don't fit nicely into a category but are considered important to comprehending the text should be added to another portion of the prereading curriculum. Once all the concepts are labeled by category, the educator develops the semantic analysis chart or semantic map. In the chart, the superordinate concept is the title, the coordinate concepts are placed along the top of the grid, and the subordinate concepts are listed along the left side of the grid (see Figure 5.1). In the map, the superordinate concept is placed in the largest circle at the top of the page (see Figure 5.2), and the coordinate concepts are placed in medium-sized circles directly attached to the superordinate concept; the subordinate concepts are placed in smaller circles attached to each coordinate concept.

When using a semantic graphic organizer as a prereading technique, it can be completed or reviewed during group instruction prior to reading the assigned material. The instructor can leave the relationship chart blank or leave off the connecting lines on the map and then guide the students to ascertain the correct relationships. In this way, the educator helps the students to use what they already know, thereby increasing their involvement with the concepts and vocabulary. The instructor also can provide a completed relationship chart or map and then review it with the students. Worksheets 5.3 and 5.4 may be used for preparing a semantic analysis chart and a semantic analysis map, respectively.

Story Grammar

A commonly used advanced graphic organizer is that of a story map. Story mapping is a graphic representation of story grammar. *Story grammar* refers to the common parts of a narrative story: the setting, characters, problems, events, and solution. In order to develop a story map, you first must read the narrative text. While reading, create a list that includes the setting, characters, problems, events, and solutions. This list is then formatted graphically (e.g., a story map). The steps are listed in Table 5.4.

(Superordinate Concept) How Fossils Are Made			
	What are fossils?	Things that can become fossils	(coordinate concept)
How we learn about dinosaurs	x		
Dinosaurs (subordinate vocabulary)		x	
Hardened tracks or footprints	x	x	
Animals or plants (subordinate idea or concept)		x	
Teeth, bones, or shells		x	

FIGURE 5.1. Example of a semantic analysis chart. Data from Bos, Anders, Filip, and Jaffe (1989).

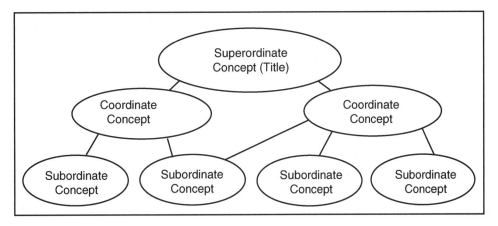

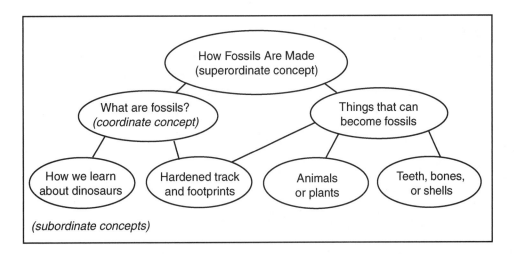

FIGURE 5.2. Example of a semantic map for an expository text. Data from Bos and Anders (1990) and based on a story from Granowsky (2000).

TABLE 5.4. Steps in Constructing Story Maps

1. Read assigned text.
2. List story grammar (i.e., characters, setting, problem, events, solutions).
3. Create graphic layout (see examples).
4. Place title for each portion of the story grammar in the desired location.
5. Place correct information in the appropriate graphic location.

Note. Data from Bos and Anders (1990).

Each part of the story grammar should be taught in a prereading exercise. When introducing these concepts, you can assist the students in looking up each part of the story. Once these parts have been taught, give students a representation of the story grammar (Bos & Anders, 1990). These graphic aids come in a variety of forms, including maps, illustrations, and charts. An example of a story grammar in chart form appears in Figure 5.3; an example of a story grammar in map form appears in Figure 5.4.

When introducing the story grammar concepts, the graphs can be given with all or some of the information provided and reviewed prior to reading. Then the students are instructed to read the story in order to confirm or disconfirm the filled-in portions of the story map and to fill in the blanks. Once a story grammar has been introduced, the graphs are usually left blank for the students to fill in while reading the story.

Choosing What Students Read

Several factors influence the type of material students should read when reading for comprehension. For example, comprehension is enhanced when students know at least 93% of the words (Hargis, 1995). This finding does not mean that harder material should be avoided entirely. In fact, in many instances, this may not be an option. Instead, the prereading procedures described earlier can be used to enhance students' knowledge of words before they are asked to read the material. Additionally, concept maps may make it simpler to comprehend material, thereby allowing the student to concentrate more on the difficult texts. Using graphic aids is particularly important when students are asked to read material that is above their instructional level.

Because fluent reading enhances comprehension, pretesting children with CBM pro-

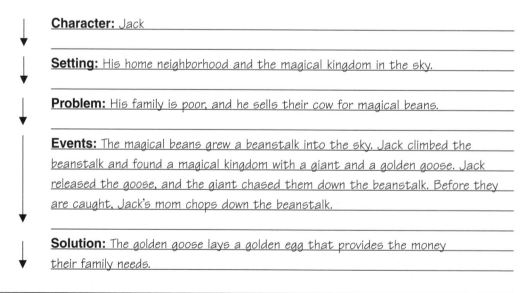

Character: Jack

Setting: His home neighborhood and the magical kingdom in the sky.

Problem: His family is poor, and he sells their cow for magical beans.

Events: The magical beans grew a beanstalk into the sky. Jack climbed the beanstalk and found a magical kingdom with a giant and a golden goose. Jack released the goose, and the giant chased them down the beanstalk. Before they are caught, Jack's mom chops down the beanstalk.

Solution: The golden goose lays a golden egg that provides the money their family needs.

FIGURE 5.3. Example of a story grammar in chart form. Data from Newby, Caldwell, and Recht (1989).

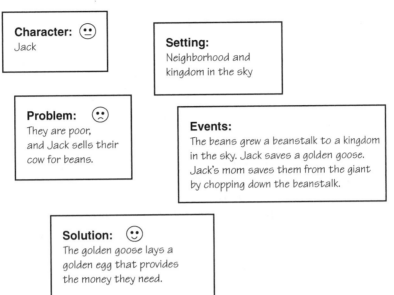

FIGURE 5.4. Example of a story grammar in map form. Data from Newby, Caldwell, and Recht (1989).

cedures (described in Chapter 4) may help you select material that is neither too difficult nor too easy. Most reading curricula are carefully designed so that passages are progressively difficult. Text length is also gradually increased. However, for students with reading skill deficits, special efforts may be needed to shape the amount of material they can read and comprehend during a particular session; for example, students can be asked to read less material than peers. You can then use shaping procedures to gradually increase the amount of material they read and the time they spend reading during a particular session (Skinner, Skinner, & Armstrong, 2000).

Students with reading skill deficits may require more time to read and comprehend material than their peers. Scanning the material, they may become discouraged by the long passages. One strategy that may help reduce frustration is to break down material into smaller units (Wallace, Cox, & Skinner, 2003). Many content area texts (e.g., science and social study books) and reading curricula break down large sections to smaller units by inserting comprehension questions, exercises, or some other activities to separate the units. With other materials, you may have to break down the material into smaller units. When reconfiguring long assignments into smaller tasks by interspersing activities, be sure that the activities are designed to enhance comprehension. Several relevant activities are described later in this chapter. Interspersing comprehension exercises more frequently may assist students who have information-processing deficits to experience more success because they are required to consolidate information from less text and over briefer intervals (Skinner, 2002). Additionally, these activities may enhance maintenance of information learned and students' ability to retrieve this information.

COMPREHENSION ACTIVITIES DURING READING

For a competent reader, comprehension of reading text can be rewarding in itself, and that reward helps to sustain the reading. Like an upward spiral, sustained reading further increases comprehension. However, students with reading problems are not likely to comprehend what they are reading, which makes sustained reading less probable. The effort involved may be one reason. We suggest, therefore, that you keep three factors in mind in this regard. First, limit distractions in the room, and if students get off-task, redirect them back to the text in a neutral but firm manner (Myerson & Hale, 1984). Second, students are more likely to engage in sustained silent reading when the teacher is also engaged in sustained silent reading (Methe & Hintze, 2003) (parents can have a similar effect at home by modeling sustained silent reading). A protocol for implementing sustained silent reading can be found in Table 5.5. The third factor to keep in mind is that breaking down large tasks into smaller tasks can help students sustain reading. For example, a 40-page chapter could be broken down into four sections by interspersing comprehension activities every 10 pages or so. Of course, section designations must comprise meaningful units; it is not helpful to divide the text in arbitrary ways. The question then becomes how to break long reading tasks into smaller, discrete sections so that there is a clear signal or cue to students that they have completed a unit. The next section describes various procedures that can be used to break long assignments into brief assignments in order to enhance, as opposed to disrupt, comprehension.

Reading Comprehension Activities

In the previous section, we discussed various forms of advanced organizers that can be used prior to reading to enhance comprehension. For students with reading skill deficits, comprehension activities that require them to answer questions or respond to the content *as they are reading* also have been shown to enhance comprehension (Robinson & Skinner, 1996).

TABLE 5.5. Protocol for Sustained Silent Reading

1. To engage in silent reading, select a time period that will have a minimum of disruption.
2. Have students select appropriate reading material (i.e., books rather than magazines or other picture-laden materials).
3. Encourage students to attend to any needs prior to beginning reading (e.g., bathroom, questions, finding nondistracting spot to read).
4. Prior to beginning reading, provide directions and a prompt to the students regarding your enjoyment of reading.
   Example: *"When I sit down, I open to where I left off and begin quietly reading every word until the bell rings. I can't wait to read what's going to happen today."*
5. Model silent reading in full view of the class for the entire allotted period.
6. Conclude the session with another prompt to the students regarding transition to the next activity, along with another comment about your enjoyment of reading.

Note. Data from Methe and Hintze (2003).

Story Grammar

Story grammar was discussed earlier as a prereading activity. These procedures also have been used as during-reading or postreading activities. While reading, students can be given a sheet of paper and asked to fill in basic information that is common to most stories (Newby, Caldwell, & Recht, 1989). Blank, reproducible worksheets for each type of story grammar (chart form and story map) appear in Worksheets 5.5 and 5.6. These worksheets prompt students to pay attention to the information necessary to understand the story. Providing students with a story grammar sheet prior to reading supplies a purpose for reading and allows students to form hypotheses about the material based on their scanning of titles, pictures, etc. Having students complete this sheet *as they read* can help them consolidate, store, and maintain information. An example of a complex story grammar related to the Jack and the Beanstalk story can be found in Figure 5.5.

Ideally, you should first teach students how to use the story grammar correctly, then observe their independent use of it, and finally, fade the use of the story grammar so that they learn how to comprehend the material unaided. Demonstration, practice, and feedback should be used to teach students the correct application of the story grammar. Students can be asked to respond to items verbally, as material is being read aloud, or by filling out worksheets as they read. Using praise, point systems, and immediate corrective

MORE COMPLEX STORY GRAMMAR QUESTIONING

1. Who is the story about? _____
   _____

2. What is the boy's job? _____
   _____

3. What problem does he have? _____
   _____

4. What does he do to try to get money for the family? _____
   _____

5. What happens when he brings magic beans home? _____
   _____

6. Where did he meet the giant? _____
   _____

7. How was the giant killed? _____
   _____

8. What happens in the end? _____
   _____

9. Could Jack have done something different to get money? _____
   _____

10. What might have happened to Jack if his mother had not cut down the stalk? _____
    _____

FIGURE 5.5. Example of a more complex story grammar in question form. Data from Grossen and Carnine (1991).

feedback encourages students to use this tool effectively. As you are fading out reliance on story grammar, students would not be given a copy of the blank story grammar form or asked to fill in their responses as they read. The teacher should still assess student comprehension, however, by asking story grammar questions after the student has finished reading (Newby et al., 1989).

Story grammars are especially effective and useful with younger students whose reading curricula are often composed of multiple simple stories that have limited characters and plots. As students' reading comprehension skills improve, story grammars can be altered to include more complex items such as (1) type of conflict (e.g., human versus nature), (2) foreshadowing (e.g., "What do you think will happen next and why do you think this?"), and (3) general themes (e.g., "Persistence helps accomplish goals").

In these examples, structured prompts or questions are provided and students are asked to respond as they read. However, students also can develop their own questions prior to reading. These self-generated questions may be particularly useful for narrative or story reading. Having students write their own questions ahead of time and then using them as guided notes may enhance overall comprehension even more than prestructured prompts (Schumaker, Deshler, Alley, Warner, & Denton, 1982). Examples of self-questions might include, "Will Johnny get caught?" and "How will he cross the bridge?"

Expository Text

As with story grammars, a variety of advanced organizers and visual graphic displays that are used to enhance comprehension of expository text prior to reading can be incorporated into reading activities. Outlines, study guides, strategic notes, time lines, and flow charts can be systematically inserted into text, and students can be instructed to answer comprehension questions as they are reading.

Outlines and Study Guides

Outlines and study guides are prepared in advance of the reading assignment and distributed to students when the reading is initially assigned. Students read the text and follow along with the outline, for example. Outlines that contain all the pertinent information can be read as a prereading activity or used as a postreading activity (e.g., as study aids). One major limitation to these procedures is that sometimes students choose to read only these summaries, as opposed to reading the text itself. Overly detailed outlines or study guides actually hinder comprehension when they discourage students from reading assigned text (McDaniel et al., 2001). With effective outlines, in contrast, students respond to items as they are reading. One example includes questions that students answer as they read. These questions are generally placed in the same sequence as the text on which they are based. Both questions and answers should be brief so as not to cause unnecessary disruptions in student reading.

Framed outlines have many similar characteristics in that prompts and responses are typically provided in the same sequence as in the text. Framed outlines are constructed

We learned about dinosaurs from their ___fossils___ . A fossil is left by a ___plant or animal___ . Fossils can be leaves, shells, ___eggs, or skeletons___ . Some fossils are the hardened tracks of ___footprints___ left by a moving ___animal___ . When an animal or plant dies, it can become covered with ___mud or sand___ . As time goes by, the plant or animal becomes covered by ___many layers___ of mud or sand. After ___thousands___ of years, the ___bottom___ layers harden into ___rock___ . The dead ___plant or animal___ also hardens into ___rock___ . This is how ___fossils___ are formed.

FIGURE 5.6. Example of a framed outline for a third-grade basal reading selection on fossils. Based on a passage from Granowsky (2000).

with brief sentences that focus on key information. Students are typically required to write brief answers. Figure 5.6 provides an example of a framed outline, in which students are required to fill in the blanks as they read (Lovitt, Rudsit, Jenkins, Pious, & Benedetti, 1986).

Strategic Note Taking

Rather than providing brief, one-word answers, students may be required to make more general notes, a technique referred to as strategic note taking (see Figure 5.7 for an example). Taking notes, however, often requires much time and energy and may end up disrupting reading. Thus, these procedures are often used with more advanced readers who can easily move back and forth from writing notes to reading. When used with less-skilled

FOSSILS

I. Fossils are left by . . .
    A.
    B.

II. Fossils can be . . .
    A.
    B.
    C.
    D.   skeletons.
    E.   hardened tracks or footprints left by a moving animal.

III. When a plant or animal dies, what happens?
    A.   It becomes covered by mud or sand.
    B.   As time goes by . . .
        1.
        2.   Dead plant or animal hardens into rock.

FIGURE 5.7. Student copy of guided note taking. Based on a passage from Granowsky (2000).

readers, these time-consuming activities are probably more appropriate at the end of the reading session.

Time Lines and Flow Charts

Two other forms of *during-reading* activities are time lines and flow charts, both of which are useful for enhancing comprehension in content areas when an understanding of linear events is important. Both forms outline the sequence of events. Time lines provide a chronological sequence of events; they help students translate narrative text by requiring them to complete summaries of events covered in the text. Figure 5.8 provides an example of a time line. Flow charts can cover chronological events or sequential physical events. For example, a flow chart might describe the sequence of blood flowing through the heart.

Conflict Charts

Conflict charts can be used during reading to aid comprehension of nonlinear concepts. With this simple procedure students are required to list support for conflicting arguments or conclusions. For example, as students are reading, they could be asked to list pros and cons of nuclear power on each side of a piece of paper. A blank, reproducible form appears in Worksheet 5.7.

Student Comprehension during Reading

Questions that outline the meaning of a text should be brief and clear to prevent major disruptions and allow students to return to reading after they answer the questions. When students are learning to use comprehension strategies while they are reading, their responses should be observable. When training groups of students to use these procedures, students can be expected to give verbal answers during recitation sessions, which allows the teacher to provide immediate, public, corrective feedback and praise so that the group can acquire these skills. When students are reading independently, they can be expected to write their answers. Writing answers has several advantages: Students can read at their own pace, independently completing answers as they progress through the exercise, and teachers can circulate around the room, evaluating, praising, and providing

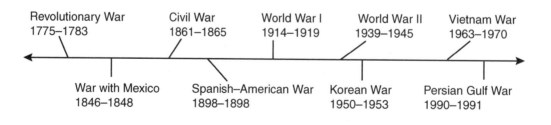

FIGURE 5.8. Example of a historical time line for U.S. wars.

corrective feedback to individual students. As a final step, prompts are faded and students are encouraged to use these comprehension strategies unaided.

Visualization

Another strategy that may enhance comprehension is that of visualization: forming a mental picture of what was read (Alesandri, 1982). Various procedures have been used to train students to use visual imagery. The simplest procedure is to tell students to form a picture in their mind (Alesandri, 1982). Pictures can be used to assist students in developing visual images (e.g., Giesen & Peeck, 1984). A story board containing a sequence of pictures may help students to develop sequential, as opposed to static, visual images (Chan, Cole, & Morris, 1990). Carnine and Kinder (1985) improved the comprehension of fourth- to sixth-grade students by asking them to make pictures in their mind of events that happened in a story as they were reading. The following day, students were encouraged to close their eyes and form images, then draw pictures of those images. Brandoof-Matter (1989) described several procedures to help students visualize. First she told students to close their eyes and picture what was being said, as material was read aloud. Then she asked them specific questions, such as, "Where are you?" (i.e., referring to the setting) and "Who is talking?" (i.e., referring to the characters). Additionally, she described an object and asked students to identify what she described.

Concluding Remarks on Comprehension Strategies Used during Reading

Although a variety of activities has been shown to be effective, some questions have yet to be answered. For example, we do not know how much material should be read independently before these activities are appropriate. A general recommendation is that with less-skilled readers, these activities should be interspersed more frequently (e.g., every page as opposed to every 10 pages). By providing less information to process before completing these activities, less-skilled readers may have more success responding accurately. Furthermore, these frequent opportunities to actively consolidate information may enhance comprehension.

It is not clear which activities are superior to others. Student perceptions of these various during-reading activities also may need to be assessed. Some students may find such activities disruptive to their reading. For example, a student who is really enjoying reading a Civil War story may not want to interrupt his or her reading to answer questions. However, for other students these disruptions may be welcome, and completing these activities may be rewarding (Skinner, 2002). Students' perceptions are critical because the goal of most of these activities is for students to implement them independently, without additional assistance or support. Students who find these activities tiresome or unhelpful are unlikely to follow the correct steps independently. Although these activities have been shown to be effective with students who have disabilities, research has not clearly identified which students are most likely to benefit. Clearly, more research is needed on during-reading comprehension enhancement procedures.

POSTREADING COMPREHENSION ACTIVITIES

After students have finished reading, a variety of procedures can by used to enhance comprehension. These include summarization and identifying the relationships between comprehension questions and the answers in the text. Students are more likely to experience success using these procedures when they apply them immediately after they have finished reading. These postreading activities also can be used to assess comprehension. Student performance on these postreading procedures provides educators with an opportunity to reinforce reading comprehension.

Summarization

When reading content area text (e.g., a science text), the goal is for students to acquire information that is needed for subsequent activities (e.g., to complete a laboratory assignment, to understand the applications of a theory, to pass an exam, to better understand subsequent reading material, lectures, or demonstrations). Summarization procedures are often used as a postreading activity to enhance comprehension and retention of expository text. Although some students may develop effective summarization skills without specific instruction, students with reading skill deficits may need to be taught these skills. For example, students have been successfully taught to write down the main ideas using their own words (Macon, 1991), organize the ideas into related groups (Fahmy & Bilton, 1990), reduce the main ideas as concisely as possible, and use an outline form to indicate main ideas and subordinate ideas (Anderman & Williams, 1986).

Nelson, Smith, and Dodd (1992) investigated the effectiveness of teaching a strategy for developing summary skills to elementary students with learning disabilities. The first seven steps focused on identifying and organizing the main ideas and important information. These steps required that students:

1. Write down the main idea.
2. Write down the important points the writer had to say about the main idea.
3. Review the text to check their understanding of the main idea and the important points related to that main idea.
4. Write down the main idea or topic that they want to write about in their summary.
5. Sequence important points (from step 2) by how they want to write about them.
6. Review the text and their notes to see if there is any important information left out or any unimportant information they can leave out.
7. Write the summary.

After written summaries were completed, the focus shifted to clarifying and revising these summaries. First, students reread their own summaries and revised them if there were any unclear points. Second, peers read each other's summaries and indicated any point that was not clear. This feedback was used to make their final revisions of the summaries. The authors of this study also provided a summary skills study guide that included the nine steps plus space to write down the requested information. Results of their study showed that this summary strategy instruction produced increases in reading comprehension scores and improved summary writing skills (Nelson et al., 1992).

Most effective summarization strategies are highly structured, and students receive specific instruction on completing their summaries. D'Alessio (1996) investigated a similar, less structured summarization strategy that incorporated a retelling technique. Students were instructed to re-create a portion of the text that they had just read or someone had read to them. Although this general procedure could easily be used across texts, D'Alessio (1996) found that merely having students retell a portion of the text, without any specific instruction as to how to re-create the text or summarize the reading, did not result in increased reading comprehension scores. Thus, it appears that students must be taught how to create summaries of text, and that the steps should be clear and structured.

Most summarization techniques have been developed to enhance comprehension of expository text. However, these techniques can be adapted for use with narrative stories. Instead of recording main ideas and grouping them by relationships, the students can be instructed to record the main character and his or her actions. These actions can be grouped by goals and relationships to other characters. Thus, students create a type of story map like the one that was described earlier in this chapter. Used in this manner, the story mapping would be considered a during- and postreading technique: The recording of main story elements occurs during reading but the relationship grouping or mapping occurs after reading has finished.

Question-and-Answer Relationship Training

Question-and-answer relationship (QAR) training is based on the idea that answering comprehension questions is not an isolated activity but one that involves a relationship between the reader, his or her background knowledge, and the text (Pearson & Johnson, 1978; Raphael, 1986). The relationships between comprehension questions and answers can be broken down into two broad categories: (1) those that are "in the book" and (2) those that the reader can answer "in my head" (Raphael, 1986). Answers to in-the-book questions are either "right there" (i.e., an explicit answer is in the text) or require a "think-and-search" procedure (i.e., an implicit answer is in the text, but the student has to find it, sometimes in multiple locations). The in-my-head questions have either author-and-you answers (i.e., an answer comes from the student, with some clues from the author) or "on-your-own" answers (i.e., the answer comes solely from within the student).

Teaching the QAR program to students follows a model–lead–test procedure. The teacher shows the students how to identify the location of the answer for a comprehension question (model). The teacher involves the students in the process of answering a comprehension question, guiding their answers (lead), and asking them for an answer (test). The students are then gradually given more independence to apply the QAR strategy to answering comprehension questions (Sorrell, 1990). In the training phase of QAR, short (e.g., between two and four sentences) text passages are used for each comprehension question. After students have acquired the skills, text passage length should be increased.

Graham and Wong (1993) improved the comprehension of fifth- and sixth-grade students by adapting the QAR program to create a simple mnemonic—the 3H strategy: "here," "hidden," and "in my head." Training for the 3H strategy is similar to the QAR program. It includes (1) modeling of the strategy (the teacher uses a think-aloud), (2) overt guidance as students apply the strategy, (3) faded self-guidance as students continue to use the strategy, and (4) covert self-instruction as the teacher withdraws assistance completely (i.e., fading).

COMBINING PROCEDURES

Some interventions combine several of the techniques already discussed and involve prereading, reading, and postreading comprehension activities. Several are reviewed next.

Strategic Note Taking

Strategic note taking can be used in all three stages of reading. Worksheet 5.8 displays a strategic note-taking form that requires students to complete sections before, during, and after reading. The top of the page provides space for the student to identify the topic of the reading material and any knowledge of that topic prior to reading. The next section instructs students to take notes in clusters or groupings as they are reading. This cue is designed to help students with organization and identification of relationships between points of information. A quick summary of the section pertaining to those key ideas is requested. The steps of clustering ideas and summarizing are repeated throughout the reading assignment. When the reading is finished, students are cued to list five main points and describe them. This postreading summarization activity provides a global overview of the entire text.

SQ3R: Survey, Question, Read, Recite, and Restate

The survey, question, read, recite, and restate (SQ3R) study approach was designed for use with expository texts (Robinson, 1946). First, students *survey* the passage, then they formulate *questions* about the titles and subheadings they read during the surveying. This step allows students to use their prior knowledge and provides a purpose for reading (i.e., to answer those questions). Next they *read* (R1) the passage for the first time. During the reading, students can answer the questions generated prior to reading either in writing, verbally, or silently. After reading, students are instructed to *recite* (R2) certain content in the passage and make notes of the answers to the questions previously generated. A final review is conducted, during which students *restate* (R3) or summarize the content (Schumaker et al., 1982).

Multipass Strategy

The Multipass strategy was developed as an improvement on the SQ3R technique (Schumaker et al., 1982). This strategy incorporates the skills of surveying, sizing up, and sorting out. Each of these skills is considered a subcategory and requires a separate pass through the text. In the first pass-through, students are asked to *survey* the text for the main ideas and the chapter organization by reading the titles, introductory paragraph, illustration captions, and the summary paragraph. Students also must review the chapter's relationship to adjacent chapters and paraphrase all the information gathered during this first pass through the text.

The second pass-through, *sizing up*, involves four steps designed to help students gain specific information from the text without reading it from beginning to end. Prior to starting the steps, students are encouraged to read the comprehension questions at the end of the chapter to see which facts appear to be the most important to remember. The steps include (a) looking for textual cues, such as bold-face print, subtitles, or italics; (b) turning the cues into a question (e.g., the subtitle cue "Civil War" might prompt the question "Who won the Civil War?" or "Who fought in the Civil War?"); (c) "skim reading" the surrounding text to answer the questions just generated; and (d) paraphrasing the answers to the questions without looking back in the book. When this pass-through is complete, readers are encouraged to paraphrase all the facts, concepts, and ideas from the chapter that they could remember.

The third and final pass-through, *sorting out*, is designed as a comprehension monitoring technique. In this step, students read all the comprehension questions at the end of the chapter. Students place a checkmark next to questions they can answer immediately and are trained to look up answers to those they don't know by using the information about text structure already gained. Once a question is answered, they place a checkmark by it.

POSSE: Predict, Organize, Search, Summarize, and Evaluate

The POSSE approach utilizes a variety of reading strategies for comprehending expository material (Englert & Mariage, 1991). POSSE is usually taught with modeling and guided learning methods. Students scan the material and then *predict* ideas based on their background knowledge; they are encouraged to brainstorm about the topic of the passage. After making their predictions, students *organize* their thoughts into a structure similar to the text; they are instructed to categorize and group ideas together (a semantic map may be used to facilitate this process). Then students begin reading and *searching* for the text structure and any cues as to text content. After reading (or intermittently), students *summarize* the main and subordinate ideas; they are encouraged to generate questions about the main ideas as they read to help facilitate the summarizing process. Finally, students *evaluate* their own comprehension by (1) comparing their summarizations and semantic maps from the *organize* section with the text, (2) clarifying any unclear points and answers to questions generated in the *summarize* section, and (3) *predicting* what will be discussed in the next section, using cues from the text or the revised semantic map.

USING REWARDS TO IMPROVE COMPREHENSION

Student performance on postreading comprehension items, questions, and tasks provides an excellent opportunity to reinforce reading and comprehension efforts. Some educators may have concerns that providing additional reinforcement for reading might reduce the intrinsic motivation for the activity. However, students with reading skill deficits and a history of failure in reading activities may need this additional reinforcement to motivate them to engage in prereading comprehension activities and to use comprehension strategies during reading (including actually reading the material) and after reading. For these reasons it is important to discuss general procedures for rewarding students' performance on postreading comprehension tasks.

First, reinforcement should be immediate and contingent upon correct performance. Initially, when teaching students specific pre-, during-, and postreading strategies, reinforcement should be delivered contingent upon correct use of the strategies themselves. Clear feedback should be given to correct any procedural errors, and students should be given an immediate opportunity to practice the steps correctly after this feedback. As students begin to use these procedures correctly, reinforcement also should be given contingent upon comprehension results. This reinforcement should include labeled praise that links the strategy to their success on a comprehension assessment (e.g., "Wow! You completed the entire strategic note-taking assignment and did great on your test!"). Finally, reinforcement for following steps correctly should be faded, while reinforcement for comprehending (e.g., a good grade on an exam) is kept in place or even strengthened to maintain comprehension. Eventually, this reinforcement also can be faded.

Although providing additional reinforcement for reading comprehension may be necessary, it is essential that the criterion for earning reinforcement be neither too difficult nor too easy. One procedure is to use very loose or randomly selected criteria (Popkin & Skinner, 2003). For example, Sharp and Skinner (in press) worked with a second-grade teacher to enhance students' reading comprehension during sustained silent reading. The teacher was using the Accelerated Reader (Renaissance Learning, 2002) program, in which students were encouraged to select material at their grade level and given time for sustained silent reading, then given additional rewards (grade enhancement and teacher praise) for passing computer-delivered exams on their text after they finished reading. Although students were allowed to choose books written at their grade level, few were passing—or even taking—the comprehension exams. Additionally, the teacher reported that many students did not appear to be reading during sustained silent reading time. The teacher and researchers wanted to develop a procedure that would encourage all students to read for comprehension. Comprehension exams would be used to assess results.

The primary concern was with how to set a criterion that would not be too high for some students (thereby causing some to give up) or too low for others (causing some to not perform their best). To solve this problem a contingency was used in which the teacher randomly selected a number (e.g., from 1 to 13) at the end of each week; if the number of exams passed by the whole class met or exceeded the chosen number for the week, the students received a group reward (e.g., watch a movie). Thus, each student was encouraged to do his or her best in order to increase the chances of the group earning their reward.

In addition, the students were told that they would all earn an ice cream party if everyone passed an exam in 6 weeks. The teacher, however, was concerned that some of the students would require additional instruction or assistance to pass an exam. The tutoring program began with students working in pairs. During sustained silent reading time (now called *quiet* reading time), pairs took turns reading aloud from the same book and discussing what was happening as they read. Peers were paired so that the two students were at the same reading level, with one exception; poor readers were paired with strong readers. These pairs took turns reading from stories written at the weaker students' reading level. After both members of the pair passed an exam, they were allowed to read on their own. Approximately half chose to continue reading in pairs, and half chose to read alone.

Results showed that whereas the class had averaged 0.7 quizzes passed per week prior to the intervention plan, it increased to 7.5 quizzes passed per week during the intervention stage. Strong readers passed many more quizzes, and weaker readers continued to read and attempt to pass quizzes. Because an interdependent group reward system was in place, the probability of earning the reward was increased when each student did his or her best. Thus, students encouraged one another to do their best and did not pester or disrupt their peers' reading.

Although this plan was successful, in many cases reinforcement for reading can be delivered in simpler ways. When students are allowed to choose what they read, a powerful and natural reward is to ask them to discuss what they have read. During these discussions, parents or teachers can ask questions about the material, but they should avoid any negative evaluation. Instead, they should encourage students' enthusiasm. Literacy circles or groups, wherein students with common interests discuss readings and share insights, can provide an excellent mechanism for peer reinforcement of reading and comprehension. Additionally, exposure to peers' insights and interpretation of literature may enhance participants' comprehension skills and appreciation of literature (Leal, 1993; Parker, Quigely, & Reilly, 1999).

ASSESSMENT

Student performance on many of the *reading* and *postreading* activities described earlier can be used to assess comprehension. Some authors who recommend using CBM probes to collect fluency data (see Chapter 4) also recommend complementing these data with comprehension assessment data collected after students have finished reading the probes (e.g., Good, Kaminski, & Smith, 2002; Shapiro, 2004a). These activities include retell procedures and answering specific questions about the passages in which assessments of reading fluency were conducted.

Oral Retell Measures of Comprehension

Story Retell

Shapiro (2004b) describes a procedure for assessing comprehension after students are finished reading stories aloud. A protocol is offered in Table 5.6. First, a story is selected that contains 150–200 words (below third-grade level) or 250–300 words (third-grade level and above). As the student reads aloud, CBM assessment procedures are applied to collect data on words correct and incorrect per minute (see Chapter 4). The assessor ceases to record errors after 1 minute, but the student continues to read aloud. After the student has fin-

TABLE 5.6. Comprehension Assessment Protocols for Story Retell

1. Select a story that contains 150–200 words (below third-grade level) or 250–300 words (third-grade level and above).
2. Have the student read the passage aloud while collecting CBM data (i.e., words correct and incorrect per minute). Stop recording errors after 1 minute, but have the student continue reading the passage aloud.
3. After finishing the passage, have the student retell the story in his or her own words (consider taping the response for ease of future scoring).
4. Record the following story elements as mentioned by the student: title, main idea, problem, goal, setting, main characters, initiating event, climax, sequence of events, solution to problem, end of story.
5. While recording, note if verbal prompts are needed during the retell process, and also note if the student was allowed to refer back to the printed story.
6. Give the student 1 point for each story element identified (problem solution and end of story receive only a half point). Prompted responses receive no points (mark with asterisk).
7. Tally the points.

Note. Adapted from Shapiro (2004b). Copyright 2004 by The Guilford Press. Adapted by permission.

ished reading, the examiner asks the student to retell the story in his or her own words. Shapiro (2004b) recommends taping the student's responses so that scoring can be completed later. While listening and relistening to the tape recording, the examiner uses a scoring sheet to note each of the following story elements mentioned by the student: title, main idea, problem, goal, setting, main characters, initiating event, climax, sequence of events, solution to problem, and end of story.

Shapiro (2004b) notes several possible variations of this assessment procedure. Specifically, the examiner can provide verbal prompts during the retell process, which are recorded on scoring sheet. Additionally, students can be asked to retell the story with or without being allowed to refer back to the printed story. Finally, rather than asking the student to read aloud, the student could be asked to read the passage silently. Regardless of which variation you choose, be consistent across assessments. If you change your procedure, you will not know whether changes in results are a function of student improvements or changes in assessment procedures. To score the student, 1 point is given for each story element, with the exception of problem solution and end of story, which receive half points. Prompted responses are noted with an asterisk, but no points are alotted.

Although the story retell procedure does provide a direct measure of reading comprehension, it has several limitations. First, it may be difficult to find stories that are both brief and contain a comprehensive plot. Although students could be asked to read longer stories, it makes this type of assessment much more time consuming (Shapiro, 2004b). Additionally, because only comprehensive stories (i.e., those with each of the story elements) can be used, the number of curricular stories available for assessment at each grade level may be reduced. Thus, procedural limitations may both increase the amount of time required to administer this form of comprehension assessment and reduce the number of available passages for assessment. More studies are needed to ensure that story retell procedures yield valid and reliable measures of comprehension. Additionally, the story retell procedure is based on accuracy only and does not include a fluency measure. Thus, it is not clear if such a procedure is sensitive enough to measure changes in students' comprehension skill development.

Retell Fluency Measure

Good et al. (2002) have developed the Retell Fluency Measure (RTM) for use with students reading from mid-first-grade to the end of third-grade levels. A protocol for RTM appears in Table 5.7. Like the story retell procedure, this assessment is administered after the student has finished a CBM probe designed to assess words correct and errors per minute. However, with this procedure students are stopped after reading aloud for 1 minute. If a student reads 10 or more words correct per minute, he or she is prompted to tell the examiner all about what was just read. As the student is speaking, the examiner records the number of words the student says. If the student pauses for 3 seconds, he or she is prompted again to "try to tell me everything you can." This prompt is given only once. The next time the student fails to talk about the passage (e.g., says nothing or talks about something else) for 5 seconds, the examiner stops the session. Otherwise the session lasts 1 minute.

Good et al. (2002) provide scoring procedures for the retell fluency measure. As long as the student appears to be retelling the current passage and not talking about something else, each word is scored, including words that are part of inaccurate or irrelevant statements. Although minor repetitions or redundancies are counted, rote repetitions and recitations are not counted in the score. When the student pauses for 3 seconds and a prompt is delivered, repeating what was said prior to the prompt does not count.

Unlike the story retell procedure, retell fluency assessment does not require the student to complete an entire story that contains all the typical components of a story (e.g., characters, conflict, problem resolution). Therefore, many brief probes can be constructed

TABLE 5.7. Comprehension Assessment Protocol for Retell Fluency

Note: This procedure may be used with students from mid-first through end of third grades.

1. Select a story that is appropriate for use as a CBM probe.
2. Have the student read aloud for 1 minute.
3. If the student read 10 or more words correct per minute, have him or her tell the examiner all about what was just read.
4. As the student speaks, the examiner records the number of words said by the student.
5. If the student pauses for more than 3 seconds, provide the following prompt: "Try to tell me everything you can." (Provide the prompt only one time.)
6. End the session when the student stops talking about the passage for 5 seconds or when 1 minute has elapsed.
7. Each word spoken about the read passage is scored as 1 point. Minor repetitions or redundancies and inaccurate or irrelevant statements are counted, but rote repetitions are not. If a prompt was given, words repeated following the prompt are not counted.
8. The assessment can continue for up to 1 minute.

Note. Based on data from Good, Kaminski, and Smith (2002).

across various forms of written material. Additionally, the assessment is timed (1 minute, maximum), perhaps yielding a more sensitive measure to changes in student performance over time. However, the criterion (i.e., number of words spoken) constitutes an indirect measure of reading comprehension, and the time required to read the material is not factored into the assessment. Additionally, although standardized administration and scoring guidelines are provided, scoring requires many rapid judgments, making it difficult to score student responses reliably.

Good et al. (2002) report a correlation of 0.59 between words retold and CBM words correct per minute. The fact that the measure of words correct per minute correlates with comprehension provides some support for this measure. However, additional research is needed that compares the story retell results (i.e., words told per minute) with performance on direct measures of reading comprehension that have strong psychometric properties (e.g., standardized measures of reading comprehension). Nevertheless, this procedure is promising because it (1) can be used across curricular materials (i.e., stories as well as expository text), (2) is brief, and (3) may be more sensitive than other measures of comprehension.

Examiner-Written Comprehension Questions

A third procedure for assessing comprehension is to construct comprehension questions based on the passage the student just read. Shapiro (2004a) recommends that examiners develop five to eight comprehension questions for CBM probes; these should include both factual and inferential questions. After the student has finished reading the passage aloud, questions are administered to assess his or her comprehension. The percent of questions answered correctly can then be used as a measure of comprehension.

There are several limitations associated with these assessment procedures when compared to the CBM reading fluency measures. Writing comprehension questions for each CBM probe will not yield the same quality of data as noting words correct per minute. Students typically do not read enough material in 1 minute to allow for the creation of a sufficient number of questions to adequately assess comprehension. Thus, the assessment can yield inaccurate or invalid data. A related concern addresses the sensitivity of the comprehension measures. When only a few questions are asked, the measure is relatively insensitive to changes in student performance (as a function of instruction). Even if 10 questions were generated for each brief probe, the range of scores still would be limited (i.e., students can only score between 0 and 100% correct). Thus, only large increments (e.g., 10%) of improvement could be measured. Additionally, a ceiling effect prevents students from scoring higher than 100% accurate.

Another limitation associated with requiring students to answer specific examiner-constructed questions is that it is extremely difficult to create questions of equal difficulty level. Thus, a student may score low on a comprehension assessment one week but higher the next week as a function of question difficulty rather than improved reading comprehension skills. Without equivalent forms, it is difficult to develop accurate and sensitive measures of comprehension that can be used to make educational decisions.

Another limitation is related to prior knowledge. Although curricular passages can be carefully constructed so that they become progressively more difficult, each student's prior knowledge is likely to influence his or her performance on comprehension questions (Pearson & Johnson, 1978). Because there is no way to measure what portion of students' success in answering comprehension questions is based on their prior knowledge, it is impossible to measure the amount of comprehension that was caused by their reading ability alone. A final limitation is that most comprehension measures do not include a measure of fluency. We turn now to an assessment strategy that does measure fluency.

Rate of Comprehension

Recently, several studies have reported use of a reading comprehension rate measure (Freeland, Skinner, Jackson, McDaniel, & Smith, 2000; Jackson, Freeland, & Skinner, 2000; McDaniel et al., 2001). A rationale for measuring *rate of comprehension* is described by Skinner, Neddenriep, Bradley-Klug, and Ziemann (2002). Imagine two students who both read the same passage and score 80% correct on comprehension questions. Also imagine one student who takes 10 minutes to read the passage and another who requires 30 minutes. If rate (i.e., time spent reading) is not incorporated into the measure of comprehension, the examiner might erroneously conclude that these students have similar reading comprehension skills. However, in fact, the student who can read quickly and understands the same amount of material has the stronger skills, is more likely to choose to read, and can understand much more material in the same amount of time.

The studies examining rate of comprehension used passages from Spargo's (1989a) *Timed Reading* series. This series contains passages from fourth-grade level to beyond high school. For each grade level, there are fifty 400-word passages, followed by 10 multiple-choice comprehension questions (five factual and five inferential). To assess comprehension rate, the examiner first has the student orally read a passage while recording the time (in minutes and seconds) required to complete the passage. Next, the student is asked the five factual and five inference questions and is not allowed to refer back to the passage. The percent of accurate answers is calculated by dividing the number of correct responses by the total number of questions (i.e., 10); this percentage provides a measure of comprehension. Then, percent of accurate answers is converted to a rate measure by dividing the percentage of questions answered correctly by the number of seconds required to read the passage. The result is multiplied by 60 seconds, yielding a measured rate of comprehension (i.e., the percent of a passage understood for each minute spent reading). A protocol for assessing rate of comprehension appears in Table 5.8.

To illustrate the uniqueness of this measure, consider two students, Freddy and Sara, who read the same passage and both answered 80% of the comprehension questions correctly. One could say they have equal comprehension levels. However, assume that Freddy only needed 2 minutes to read the passage, whereas Sara needed 8 minutes. In this instance, Freddy's comprehension percentage-per-minute score would be 40% per minute, indicating that he understood 40% of the passage for each minute spent reading. However, Sara's comprehension per minute would be only 10%.

TABLE 5.8. Protocol for Rate of Comprehension Assessment

1. Select a passage containing approximately 400 words. Create 10 multiple-choice questions for that passage, five of which are factual and five of which are inferential.
2. Have the student orally read the passage while recording the time required to complete it.
3. Have the student answer the 10 questions without referring back to the passage.
4. Calculate the percent of accurate answers by dividing the number correct by the total number of questions.
5. Convert percent of accurate answers to rate by dividing the percentage of accurate answers by the number of seconds required to read the passage.
6. Multiply that number by 60 seconds to determine the percent of passage understood for each minute spent reading.

Converting comprehension accuracy to a rate measure based on time required to read the material may provide a more sensitive, direct, and educationally valid measure of comprehension skill development than merely measuring accuracy on comprehension questions (Skinner et al., 2002). However, there are important limitations to this method. As with comprehension accuracy, rate of comprehension is still influenced by a student's prior knowledge as well as by degree of question difficulty. Additionally, this method requires students to read text of the same length and difficulty level (i.e., same number of words, written at the same reading level). Thus, in most instances, such procedures cannot employ the students' reading curricula, unless oral reading results are first converted to words correct per minute. Furthermore, it is not yet clear whether students should read aloud or silently during these assessments. Finally, as with other measures of comprehension, additional research is needed to establish the sensitivity, validity, and reliability of measures of reading comprehension rate (Skinner et al., 2002).

Cautious Decision Making Based on Comprehension Assessment

Although the measure of words correct per minute correlates with reading comprehension, researchers who recommend using CBM oral reading fluency probes usually also recommend performing some sort of comprehension assessment procedure. There are several reasons for this added recommendation. First, although group studies show a strong correlation between oral reading fluency and reading comprehension, in some students this correlation may be weak. One concern is with *word callers*—that is, students who can read rapidly but fail to comprehend (Shapiro, 2004a). A second concern is with face validity. Regardless of the strong support for reading fluency as a measure, many educators are not comfortable with using an indirect measure of reading comprehension (Good et al., 2002). A final concern is that correlations between CBM oral reading fluency measures and standardized measures tend to become weaker as students progress beyond the third-grade reading level (Skinner et al., 2002). Thus, words correct per minute may not provide a very sensitive, reliable, or valid measure of reading skills in more advanced readers.

Another concern is that repeated measurement of oral reading fluency may encourage the wrong attitude about reading. For example, one of us (C.H.S.) used CBM procedure to assess a high school student's progress. Each week the student received a probe. Additionally, the student was provided feedback with respect to words correct per minute; his progress was shown to him on a graph. After a few weeks the student changed his behavior during the probes. Specifically, as the examiner read the instructions, the student took a deep breath. As the stopwatch was started and the student was told to begin reading, he began spewing out the passage, reading very rapidly, disregarding punctuation or inflection. It is possible that the CBM procedure encouraged this type of reading, and words correct per minute on these probes bore little relation to the student's reading skill development, especially reading in the area of comprehension.

The comprehension assessment activities described above can be used as a broad gauge of students' comprehension of the specific material that they have just read. For example, Good et al. (2002) report that student retell scores are typically 50% of their words correct per minute score. They suggest a rough rule of thumb: When a student's retell score is less than or equal to 25% his or her words correct per minute, this measure (i.e., words correct per minute) may not provide an accurate measure of overall reading skills.

Although we encourage assessment of reading comprehension, we also agree with Good et al. (2002) and Shapiro (2004a) that assessment results should be used with caution. Although results provide some general indication of comprehension skills, much more research is needed before any important educational decisions (e.g., where to place a student in the curriculum, whether to alter reading interventions) can be based solely on these assessment probes. Instead, such assessments may be used for screening or to supplement other assessment methods that have been shown to be valid, reliable, and sensitive (e.g., words correct per minute, standardized reading comprehension scores).

CONCLUDING COMMENTS ON COMPREHENSION STRATEGIES

Researchers have described processes and variables that cause strong readers to become better readers, while weak readers fall farther and farther behind their peers (Skinner, 1998; Stanovich, 1986; Wong, 1986). Whereas explanations differ according to theoretical models, one point they all have in common is that *reading skills improve when students read*. Thus, as students progress to the stage where comprehension is the primary reading target, it is critical that all involved encourage students to read. This is especially true for students with reading deficits who require more time and effort to read and comprehend.

WORKSHEET 5.1. TELLS Worksheet

WHAT IS THIS STORY ABOUT?

Title What is the title of this story? Does it give a clue as to what the story is about? What do you think it is about?

_____

_____

_____

Examine Look at each page of the story to find clues about the story. What did you find?

_____

_____

_____

_____

Look Look for and write down important words, such as ones that are bold or used frequently. What do they mean?

_____

_____

_____

_____

Look Look again through the story for hard words—words you do not know. Write them down. What do they mean?

_____

_____

_____

_____

Setting Write down clues about the setting, such as the place, date, and time period. (Hint: These clues are often found in the beginning of the story.)

_____

_____

_____

_____

FACT or FICTION? Is this a true story (fact)? Or is this a pretend story (fiction)?

_____

_____

_____

_____

WORKSHEET 5.2. Preteaching Unknown Words

WHAT DOES IT MEAN?

Directions: Make a list of words you do not know. Then write a definition for each word. The definition can be another word that means the same thing or a short description of that word.

Word   Definition

WORKSHEET 5.3. Preparing a Semantic Analysis Chart

Topic: _____

List the key concepts and vocabulary:

_____

_____

_____

_____

_____

_____

_____

_____

_____

Create the semantic analysis chart:

1. Find the all-inclusive idea, which becomes the title of the graph (superordinate concept).
2. Organize the concepts and vocabulary into categories (e.g., characteristics, steps, examples, functions).
3. Each main concept becomes a coordinate concept, the next step on the graph (second, third, and fourth columns).
4. Supporting concepts and vocabulary for each coordinate concept become the subordinate concepts, the final step on the graph (down first column).
5. Fill in the relationships between coordinate and subordinate concepts by marking them with an X.

WORKSHEET 5.4. Preparing a Semantic Analysis Map

Topic: _____

List the key concepts and vocabulary:

_____

_____

_____

_____

_____

_____

_____

_____

Create the semantic analysis map:

1. Identify the all-inclusive idea, which becomes the title of the map (superordinate concept; largest circle).
2. Organize the concepts and vocabulary into categories (e.g., characteristics, steps, examples, functions).
3. Each main concept becomes a coordinate concept, the next level on the map (medium circle).
4. Supporting concepts and vocabulary for each coordinate become the subordinate concepts, the final level on the map (smallest circles).
5. Fill in the relationships between coordinate and subordinate concepts by connecting them with lines.

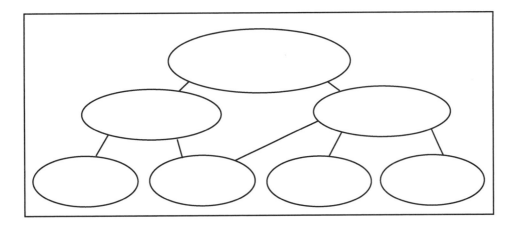

WORKSHEET 5.5. Story Grammar in Chart Form

Name: _____

Story Title: _____

    ↓   Characters: _____

           _____

    ↓   Setting: _____

           _____

    ↓   Problems: _____

           _____

    ↓   Events: _____

           _____

           _____

           _____

           _____

    ↓   Solution: _____

           _____

WORKSHEET 5.6. Story Grammar in Mapping Form

Name: _____

Story Title: _____

Characters: 😐

Setting:

Problems: ☹️

Events:

Solution: 😊

WORKSHEET 5.7. Conflict Chart

Student Name: _____

Topic: _____

Pro (Arguments in support of)	**Con** (Arguments against)

WORKSHEET 5.8. Strategic Note-Taking Form

Student Name: _____

Before reading, answer the following:

What is today's topic? Describe what you know about the topic.

_____
_____
_____

As you read, answer the following:

New Vocabulary or Terms:

_____
_____

Name three to seven main points about today's topic as they are discussed.

1. _____
2. _____
3. _____
4. _____
5. _____
6. _____
7. _____

Quickly summarize how these ideas are related.

_____
_____

New Vocabulary or Terms:

_____
_____

Name three to seven main points about today's topic as they are discussed.

1. _____
2. _____
3. _____
4. _____
5. _____
6. _____
7. _____

(continued)

Quickly summarize how these ideas are related.

_____

_____

New Vocabulary or Terms:

_____

_____

Name three to seven main points about today's topic as they are discussed.

1. _____
2. _____
3. _____
4. _____
5. _____
6. _____
7. _____

Quickly summarize how these ideas are related.

_____

_____

At the end of reading, answer the following:

Write five main points of the lecture and describe each point.

1. _____

_____

2. _____

_____

3. _____

_____

4. _____

_____

5. _____

_____

6

Accountability

The Measure of Professional Performance

We assume that at least part of your professional motivation is to make a tangible difference in the lives of your clients. We also assume (reasonably, we think) that you have been reading this book to try to get new ideas about how you can have a greater impact on those you serve. You want to *see* a difference as a result of your efforts. Regardless of whether that's a correct assumption or not, we are 100% sure that you at least want or need *someone else* to see a difference. Otherwise, the client won't come back for help and you may be out of business. You will judge the value of this book according to whether it truly helps you get results. An essential part of *getting* results, however, is how you go about *finding* them. An archeologist who does an amazing restoration of an ancient site but who provides the wrong map to get to the site can't effectively share the results of his or her work, and others cannot benefit from it. You may make productive changes in reading instruction, but if you are not monitoring and evaluating the right areas (the road map for telling whether you are getting where you are going), you won't see the improvements. On the other hand, you might change what you are doing in an *un*productive way. For instance, you might put a complex intervention in place, but the intervention is no more effective than what was being done in the first place. Here, too, if you are not monitoring the right areas, you will not see the need for other changes and will probably burden an already overloaded school system—be it a classroom, school, or district.

Our objective in this chapter is to help you create a road map for conveying the outcomes of the types of services you deliver, regardless of the scope of those services (e.g., individual consulting services, a multidisciplinary intervention team, a building-wide reading program, a district-level plan for reading intervention services). Services that are accountable are more likely to be (1) effective and (2) sought out in the future. The fields of education and psychology increasingly recognize this simple truth. Changes in these fields are also occurring because of pressures that societal forces, such as the federal government and taxpayers, bring to bear on education. Our practices are being scrutinized more than ever. For these reasons, assessment has been a dominant theme throughout this book. Assessment information should tell you whether changes are effective; such information is especially useful when it points to the types of changes you can make in the future. That is why we have concentrated on assessment methods that are direct and straightforward (i.e., don't involve leaps of inference or obscure theoretical propositions) and that facilitate ongoing monitoring of classroom or tutoring modifications. However, if you apply the model promoted in this book, you will likely accumulate a diverse collection of intervention cases, with some data for each client (with baseline and intervention phases for each case). Although these data may have helped you along the way, with each individual case, the larger question is how effective your interventions have been across *all* of the cases you have handled. You may want to know this answer by way of evaluating your effectiveness as a consultant, or perhaps you want to evaluate a new reading program that has been put in place in a school building or a district.

This chapter is meant to guide you in this process of evaluating outcomes beyond the individual case. Fortunately, there is not a lot of additional work, as you will be able to use the rich database that you have already generated from your individual cases to examine effectiveness more broadly. First, we review why accountability is fundamental to success and tie it to emerging educational innovations for addressing reading problems. Next, we present a model of accountability that should help you to organize the reporting of your service delivery results. Use of the model is demonstrated to get you started in documenting your effectiveness across cases. Finally, we share some concluding thoughts about putting all the pieces together.

THE IMPORTANCE OF ACCOUNTABLE PRACTICE

For many years and in many professional circles, effectiveness of psychological services was determined based on expert opinion. After all, the psychologist was the one who had the professional training in detecting and treating psychological disorders. Determination of effectiveness was reserved to "clinical judgment," which has had a hallowed status in the profession of psychology. Recently, however, society and the profession itself have woken up to the fact that expert judgments are still subjective, even if they are made by professionals. Indeed, psychologists had a material interest in being the ones who could identify pathology and in pronouncing their success at treating it. This gave them special status and legitimacy in the eyes of the public. The problem is that no amount of professional training guarantees objectivity. Cone (2001) stated, "We know, for example, that clinicians (and scientists, too, for that matter) tend to adopt a confirmatory approach to testing their understanding of a particular client. That is, they form early hypotheses about the client's problems and go about recruiting evidence to support those hypotheses" (p. 9). In other words, professionals tend to find what they are looking for in the first place, while ignoring data that fail to support, or may even contradict, preferred hypotheses (Dawes, 1995). If they wanted to find their services effective, the standard reliance on clinical judgment was a likely means of guaranteeing an evaluation of positive outcomes. In this age of dwindling resources, our constituents are likely to be more skeptical than we are about the value of our services in light of the cost of those services.

Overcoming Sources of Professional Error in Practice

Making data-based judgments is a step in the right direction, but it is not a panacea if a rigorous approach is not taken. Even when judgments of effectiveness are based on assessment data, there is still room for error. Although some tests are better than others, there is *always* some error in our measurements. Often, psychologists claim that through clinical judgment they can overcome that error. Their thinking goes something like the following: "Well, I'm an objective and well-trained professional. I can overcome the limitations of the assessment techniques because my finely honed clinical skills can rise above the weaknesses of the techniques I use." Unfortunately, half a century of research on professional judgment does not support this view and, on the contrary, clearly indicates that professionals *cannot* improve upon the quality of assessment information through clinical judgment. In a review of the research in this area, Dawes (1994) pointed out that professionals are only as accurate as the techniques they use, and that professional experience does not increase accuracy at all. Therefore, the decisions made based on assessment information are only as good as the quality of the assessment information itself. This conclusion is humbling for those of us who like to think that our professional experience somehow makes us more qualified than the average layperson to determine effectiveness. Frankly, it represents wrong thinking. Our job should be to *show* the layperson how we are effective (*when* we are effective) through high-quality data and to *modify* our activities when we are not effective. We haven't fulfilled our responsibility to society, the community, and our clients if (1) we can't objectively show what's working, and (2) we are unresponsive or defensive and territorial about an effective intervention plan.

The Need for Local Validation of Outcomes for Professional Services

Changes in professional attitudes about the importance of choosing evidence-based treatments reflect this trend toward accountable practice. A couple of developments are noteworthy in this respect. Two divisions of the American Psychological Association—Divisions 12 and 16—have developed coding manuals for identifying effective interventions that have appeared in the research literature (Division 16's coding manual can be accessed online at *http://www.wp-ebi.org*). Making use of these coding manuals will help the respective fields of clinical and school psychology to identify and disseminate interventions that are likely to be effective. In the field of education, the U.S. Department of Education's Institute of Education Sciences has created the "What Works Clearinghouse" (available online at *http://w-w-c.org/*) to provide an independent and objective database for effective educational interventions in areas such as beginning reading instruction, effective math instruction, adult literacy, and a host of other topics. All of these examples point to the fact that standards for the quality of interventions expected by the public in the areas of education and mental health are increasing; interventions are expected to be scientifically sound. These developments are very exciting and have potential for improving literacy, as practitioners and clients become more knowledgeable about evidence-based and scientifically sound interventions.

There is a caveat to the use of widely disseminated knowledge bases for selecting empirically valid interventions. Just because an intervention has been shown to be effective in research studies does not guarantee that it will work for your clients. If you choose a scientifically sound intervention, the chances are perhaps greater that the intervention will work. However, it is your professional responsibility to *show* that it works. In other words, you choose a valid intervention, and then you must validate it for the client. We refer to this latter process as *local validation* of a client-centered intervention. This concept also applies to the range of services you deliver when you consider all the clients that you or your program serves. Table 6.1 displays three related questions that point to the heart of accountability for the reading intervention approach adopted in this book. These questions should serve as the guiding framework for stimulating local validation of services across clients.

The first question, "How do you gauge your effectiveness across cases?", is important from a professional development perspective (Cone, 2001). As noted earlier, experts could not be more wrong when they assume that their many hours of experience render them effective. *Effective* experts monitor their performance and take a more skeptical attitude about the quality of their services prior to intervention and validation of outcome. Also, they regularly monitor effectiveness during intervention and adjust practices according to the data after intervention. The second question raises the problem of summarizing results across cases when planned modifications and monitoring have been done on a case-by-case basis. How do you evaluate your impact on the intervention-based model you have adopted when cases may be so different from one another? Finally, the third question acknowledges that the scope of intervention efforts varies from situation to situation. Some readers work as individual consultants who want to examine their personal, professional effectiveness. Other readers implement and administer reading intervention plans in one or more schools or perhaps even throughout an entire district. Some readers work as individual consultants while aspiring to expand efforts to serve more students in a building, a program, or a district. The evaluation model described in this chapter is applicable to all these scenarios. It is also flexible in that it allows for expansion of services, thereby meet-

---

TABLE 6.1. Questions Stimulating Cross-Case Accountability

- How do you gauge your effectiveness across cases?
- How do you demonstrate the value of your service when it is based primarily on individualized child studies, with each case being different from another?
- How do you demonstrate accountability at the individual level, at the building level, at the program level, at the district level?

---

ing the needs of this last group. The model intersects well with whatever organizational level and scope you wish to target, all the way from the "Lone Ranger" who is fearlessly helping to solve reading problems on a case-by-case basis to those implementing district-level programs.

The Changing Context for Meeting the Needs of Students with Reading Problems

Before we move on to a description of the components and use of the model, we want to point out one more reason why accountability is so important and explore its implications for the current context of reading assessment and intervention. Until recently, psychologists who conducted assessments were largely concerned with the psychometric properties of the tests they administered. The psychometric properties basically boiled down to how well the test correlated with itself under various conditions and how well it correlated with other known measures of the same factor. The various types of correlation and other forms of test data analysis relate to the empirical reliability and validity of the tests. Although these concerns were important, the perspective remained incomplete until Messick (1995) helped the field to understand the critical need for examination of the *social consequences* of testing and assessment. Whenever educators and psychologists conduct assessments, there are potential social consequences for the students. Obviously, if the social consequences are not positive, then the whole enterprise is questionable. If the consequences are neutral (i.e., there are no real positive or negative consequences for students), then districts and taxpayers have wasted money on unnecessary testing (and the ultimate outcome is not really so neutral). If the consequences are bad, then they not only wasted money, but they also harmed the very students they are serving! This is why it is so essential to consider issues such as testing bias and minority overrepresentation in special education programs. Barnett and Macmann (1992) reduced both of these issues to two questions:

1. What can be said with confidence (i.e., the psychometric properties)?
2. What can be said that might be helpful (i.e., the social consequences)?

These questions set the standard according to which services should be judged; they should be applied to every database that is used for any decision we make about our clients (Barnett, Lentz, & Macmann, 2000).

To demonstrate that these are not just theoretical issues of limited practical significance, we look briefly at how the field has been identifying reading disabilities and some of the major changes that have begun to emerge because of a more critical attitude about the quality of services available to students with reading disabilities. Any change in the field's approach to identifying learning disabilities has serious implications for how *you* address the needs of students with reading problems and how you justify your approach in relation to meeting their needs (the accountability aspect). *Specific learning disability* is the largest category of students with disabilities in federally funded programs. No fewer than 45.7% of all students with disabilities were classified as having "specific learning disabilities" in the year 2000 (the most recent statistics are available on the NCES website: *http://nces.ed.gov/ edstats/*). There seems to be consensus that about 80% of all students with learning disabilities have a reading disability (National Research Council, 1998). These figures represent a very large number of students with recognized problems; and they don't even account fully for *all* students who have reading problems. For instance, many students classified as behaviorally disordered also have reading and other academic problems (Lane, Gresham, & O'Shaughnessy, 2002).

Whether we like it or not, our practices reflect a model that we adopt either explicitly or implicitly. The implementation of the model is precisely where the question of consequences for students is played out in the schools. In the field of learning disabilities, the dominant model for identifying students as learning disabled has been categorical in nature and based on a significant and severe discrepancy between IQ tests and achievement tests. This model has come under heavy fire because of unreliability, questionable validity of the practice on various grounds (e.g., an inability to discriminate between experiential and cognitive bases of disability), and questionable treatment outcomes for students once they are identified (Kavale & Forness, 1999; Macmann & Barnett, 1999; Vellutino, Scanlon, & Tanzman, 1998). This is a case where a widespread assessment and diagnostic practice (1) could not inspire confidence in its own results, and (2) has not proven helpful to the students to whom the model was being applied.

To redress the problem of poor outcomes for students labeled by the categorical, discrepancy-based learning disabilities model, there is a move in the field of learning disabilities to conceptualize the problem in a radically different way. Numerous researchers are advocating a *treatment-based approach* to identifying disabilities (Fuchs & Fuchs, 1998; Fuchs, Fuchs, & Speece, 2002; Gresham, 2001; Vellutino et al., 1998; Vaughn, Linan-Thompson, & Hickman, 2003), wherein a series of interventions is first tried and monitored before a student is placed in special education. The most carefully operationalized version of this model is one in which students receive increasingly intense services if they fail to demonstrate both an adequate level of performance *and* adequate growth over time (Fuchs & Fuchs, 1998; Fuchs et al., 2002; Speece & Case, 2001). By successively implementing a series of carefully monitored interventions, practitioners directly determine (1) whether they have confidence in the results, and (2) whether their services are actually helpful by conducting ongoing evaluation, validation, and adjustment in response to results achieved with each intervention. Fuchs and colleagues (2002) go a step further and challenge practitioners to demonstrate the value of special education *before* eligibility is determined. This model of validation should still apply (and with all the more reason) once a student has become eligible for services because of a severe problem. This shift in approach illustrates how the field is being called on to take responsibility for outcomes by directly monitoring students' responsiveness to intervention. The model and practices presented in this book fit in well with this "response-to-intervention" approach in which (1) educators are accountable for each phase of service delivery (i.e., treatments are validated locally), and (2) intensity of intervention is increased when students are unresponsive to simpler interventions (i.e., services are delivered until an effective treatment is identified).

ROUNDING OUT YOUR READING INTERVENTION-BASED SERVICES WITH AN ACCOUNTABILITY COMPONENT

An Explicit Model of Service Delivery

When students are referred to you or your reading program, what can stakeholders (i.e., parents, teachers) expect of you? What exactly will you do? What common factors, issues, or characteristics span your cases, despite the different circumstances that lead up to each referral? How can you justify your professional preferences, choices, and actions relative to other methods you could be employing to address the problems? How do you respond to legal, ethical, and professional mandates for best practice? How can you demonstrate all the reasons for your choices to those you serve as well as to your colleagues? These questions point to the importance of having an explicit and justifiable model of service delivery. Inadequate answers to any of these questions mean that the services provided (1) are not standard across clients (which will lead to varying outcomes across clients), (2) cannot be justified to constituents and other professionals, and (3) may not be an efficient and productive use of anyone's time.

An Explicit Model of Accountability

As we saw in the case of identifying reading disabilities, the first step demonstrating your accountability is substantiating the validity of the model you apply to reading referrals. This means that you need to describe those procedures that you follow for each and every case (i.e., standard services). Going through this process forces you to think through why these procedures are necessary and how they relate to the overall objectives of your program and the priorities of the setting in which you work. This kind of planning is likely to improve your efficacy. Furthermore, each case comes with ethical and legal obligations, which you fulfill (or not). You had better be prepared to describe what you do and explain how your procedures help you to meet your ethical and legal responsibilities when questions come up (and they will!).

The next step in demonstrating accountability involves careful documentation of the specifics of each case. Who was served? Why? How long? By whom? What exactly was done? These questions relate to the implementation of services. The final broad area of accountability is that of client outcomes. Since you probably have multiple clients, you need to be able to summarize results across those cases to show the broad impact of the standard services you provide (beyond the individual child findings). You need methods for quantifying those outcomes for when people say "Show me!" These three areas of accountability are summarized in Table 6.2.

The first item in Table 6.2 refers to a procedural checklist, which is the operational definition of your service delivery model. Such a checklist outlines the steps that you take with each and every case (despite peculiarities and differences across cases) and serves as a communication tool for explaining how you serve clients; it holds those responsible for the services accountable for key aspects of the model in every case (Barnett et al., 1999). A sample 10-item procedural checklist can be found in Worksheet 6.1 (all worksheets are at

TABLE 6.2. An Evaluation Model for Data-Based Consultation and Intervention Services

- Requires an explicit model for service delivery that is described in a procedural checklist.
- Requires documentation of the services implemented.
- Produces a quantitative synthesis across sources of information (data).

the end of the chapter). The circumstances of your service delivery (e.g., individual consultant vs. a member of a problem-solving team) will create slightly different priorities. The example in Worksheet 6.1 describes the minimal procedural steps necessary for conducting adequate problem solving. A checklist that addresses all your legal, ethical, organizational, and professional requirements should be developed prior to services. In cases where a team approach is used, this step can serve as a very useful collaborative exercise for achieving agreement among members about exactly what assessments and interventions will be administered with each case. The checklist should be filled out for each case and filed with other data on an ongoing basis. The results will tell you whether the minimal, standard steps are being followed for each case. If all the steps are followed routinely but outcomes are disappointing, then you know that your model needs to be changed in some way. If the steps are not followed routinely, then you know that there is inconsistency in service delivery.

The procedural checklist constitutes one source of data that indicates whether the overall model is being implemented consistently, as planned. For individual cases, the percentage of steps completed can be calculated by dividing the number of steps completed (e.g., 9 steps) by the total number of steps on the checklist (10 in the example; producing a score of 90%). Descriptive statistics such as mean, median, range, and standard deviation can be reported to give an indication of how consistently the model is implemented. This source of data ("procedural integrity") is one of the multiple data sources cited in Table 6.3. When summarized with other types of data, and when the results are consistently high across data sources, you have converging, supportive evidence that indicates the impact of your services on clients.

TABLE 6.3. Means of Synthesizing Various Sources of Data

- Procedural integrity (procedural checklist)
- Effect size
- Percentage of nonoverlapping data
- Goal-attainment scaling
- Treatment integrity (i.e., fidelity and consistency)
- Social validity

Data Summarization Methods

The accountability model requires repeated assessments conducted across time for each case—the basic model for assessment that has been presented in this book. These assessment results are the child outcomes that can be summarized and synthesized via the other techniques that appear in Table 6.3. Each of the data summary methods has advantages and disadvantages, and no single method is sufficient, in itself, to evaluate service quality. Combined, however, they can give an overall indication of consultant or program effectiveness. Each is discussed in turn.

Effect Size

Although this sounds like a complicated and intimidating statistic, effect sizes are computationally simple and not particularly difficult to interpret. Indeed, they have become so important that the American Psychological Association requires that they be reported in its journals (American Psychological Association, 2001). Effect sizes can be calculated for studies and for individual cases that have repeated measures of baseline and intervention phases. A collection of cases that each has one or more effect sizes can be summarized by reporting the descriptive statistics (i.e., means, medians, ranges, and standard deviations). First, let's start with what an effect size means (no pun intended). For individual cases, the effect size describes where the average intervention data point stands in the distribution of baseline data. Imagine that you didn't do anything for the client; you just measured his or her performance repeatedly over a brief period of time (before new learning could occur). You would get some variability in the results because of error and irrelevant differences from one assessment to the next. However, with a good measure, the results should cluster around an average in somewhat of a normally distributed manner (like the bell curve you see in statistics books).

Now, fast forward to when you have actually intervened and have enough data points (e.g., 7–10) to evaluate the treatment. You would expect those data points in the baseline (no intervention) distribution to be higher than most of the baseline data points. Right? An effect size tells you where the average intervention data point stands in the distribution of baseline data points. For an academic skill such as reading, you would expect the difference between the intervention mean and the baseline mean to be a positive number (i.e., intervention mean − baseline mean > 0). An effect size merely describes that difference in standard deviation units. The standard deviation expresses the average amount of variability in the distribution of scores. This figure is important because different types of scores will produce larger or smaller differences, making it impossible to compare across scores without some means of standardizing results. Because the effect size is described in standard deviation units, it standardizes *all* reporting of effect sizes. This way, you can compare effect sizes across completely different measures. The larger the effect size, the stronger the treatment. Cohen's (1988) guidelines for effect sizes are often cited to assist with interpretation: An effect size of 0.20 is considered *small*; an effect size of 0.50 is considered *moderate*; and an effect size of 0.80 or greater is considered *large*. An effect size of +1.0 means that the average intervention data point stands one standard deviation above the baseline mean (this is good for skilled behaviors such as reading); an effect size of –1.0 means that the average intervention data point stands one standard deviation below the baseline mean (this is bad for skilled behaviors such as reading—it means that things are getting worse rather than better). Kratochwill, Elliott, and Busse (1995) argue that an effect size of +1.0 or greater represents a clinical and practical change of significant magnitude.

Although there are a number of different computational formulas for calculating effect sizes, and statisticians debate the virtues of each method, a simple approach that makes no assumptions about underlying distributions of scores and is appropriate for individual case work data is described here (Busk & Serlin, 1992). The formula and an example appear in Figure 6.1. You can see the corresponding graph of the data. As noted earlier, the mean of the baseline data is subtracted from the mean of the intervention data, and the result is divided by the baseline standard deviation. In the example in Figure 6.1, the effect size is quite large relative to conventional standards. This large effect size corresponds with the clear, visible increase in trend during the intervention phase. If you are already sweating about the calculations, we will share some information that will make it much easier for you: There is a website that will do all the computational work for you. At *http://www.interventioncentral.org*, the "Chart Dog" tool (under the "Tools for Educators" link) will plot your data on a graph (sweet, huh!), and you can ask it to calculate an effect size for each chart that you make.

Percentage of Nonoverlapping Data

Here's another statistic with an intimidating name that betrays a deceptively simple idea. One way to figure out whether there has been a difference between baseline and intervention is to calculate the percentage of data points that are higher than the highest baseline data point. Although not as elegant or as robust as the effect size, the percentage of nonoverlapping data (PND) is a simple summary statistic that is easy to calculate. You will find an example in Figure 6.2 for the same graph that was used in the effect size example. In all, there are 12 intervention data points, and 11 of those data points are higher than 38 (the highest baseline data point). Therefore, the statistic is computed, in this case, as 11/12, or 92%. PND is especially useful when you cannot calculate effect sizes; you won't be able to calculate effect sizes when you have a standard deviation of 0 (i.e., undefined; a rare occurrence) or when you have fewer than two baseline data points (because you won't be able to calculate a standard deviation). We suggest that you use PND as a backup for the few cases where you can't calculate effect sizes. The "Chart Dog" feature at *http://www.interventioncentral.org* will also calculate PND for you. (Isn't this getting easier all the time?)

Goal-Attainment Scaling

Goal-attainment scaling is a method for quantifying judgments of overall treatment effectiveness. After considering the circumstances of the case, the outcome data, and the degree to which the client achieved (or failed to achieve) goals, you assign a number to the

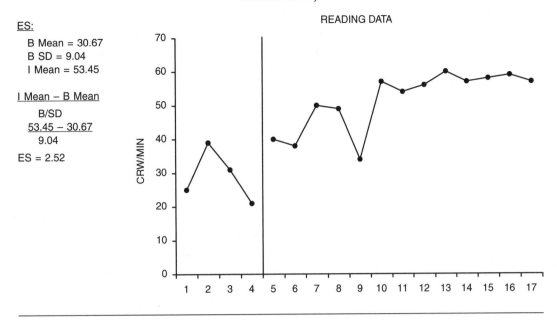

ES:
  B Mean = 30.67
  B SD = 9.04
  I Mean = 53.45

I Mean − B Mean
  B/SD
  53.45 − 30.67
  9.04
ES = 2.52

FIGURE 6.1. An example of calculating an effect size.

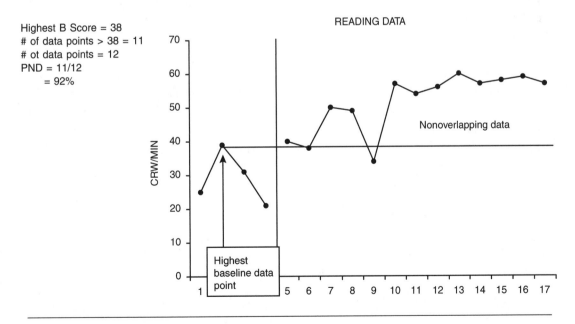

Highest B Score = 38
# of data points > 38 = 11
# ot data points = 12
PND = 11/12
     = 92%

FIGURE 6.2. An example of calculating the percentage of nonoverlapping data.

case. A higher number means that greater goal attainment was achieved, a *0* means that no progress was made toward the goal, and a negative number means that things got worse rather than better for the client. The larger the negative number, the worse things got after treatment.

Goal-attainment scaling is commonly used in consultation research. For instance, Kratochwill et al. (1995) used goal-attainment scaling when they reported the effects of training 17 school psychology graduate students in behavioral consultation. The trainees engaged in case-centered consultation that involved problem solving, continuous progress monitoring, and data-based decision making (much like the model presented in this book). The trainees served as consultants on multiple cases. Cases were rated based on reports, effect sizes, and graphs on a scale from +2 to –2. Definitions for ratings appear in Table 6.4. In all, there were 44 cases. Several cases were terminated early for various reasons, so goal-attainment scaling ratings were made in 37 cases. The researchers found that the behavioral goal was fully met (+2) for 11 cases and partially met (+1) for 19 cases. For 6 cases there was no progress toward the goal (0), and for 1 case the behavior was somewhat worse.

In a similar evaluation of consultant training outcomes, Barnett et al. (1999) used a goal-attainment scale from +2 to –2. The median goal-attainment scaling rating was +1 (range, –1 to +2). The results indicated that 42% of the cases fully met their goal (+2), 42% partially met their goal (+1), 14% did not make progress toward the goal (0), and 2% (i.e., 1 case) was somewhat worse after services (rated as –1). These reports are instructive for two reasons. First, the results for goal-attainment scaling and the other measures they used (e.g., effect sizes, PND, procedural checklists) clearly indicate that services were effective in most cases. Therefore, those pursuing data-based consultation service delivery should be encouraged. Additionally, the researchers demonstrate how to summarize results across cases when the cases are individualized (to meet clients' needs) and target very different factors. Essentially, each case is a kind of mini-experiment in itself, in which the same flexible model is applied.

If you follow the model presented in this book, you will have the database to generate goal-attainment scaling ratings. We suggest a five-step procedure (see Table 6.5). First, look for objective, independent, but knowledgeable professionals who can serve as raters for your cases. After you have collected a number of cases (e.g., at the end of the year), tell the raters that you will take them out to lunch if they will read your case summaries and rate them. Second, we suggest that you have multiple raters evaluate cases at one time.

TABLE 6.4. Goal-Attainment Scaling Definitions for Ratings

- +2 = behavioral goal fully met
- +1 = behavioral goal somewhat met
- 0 = no progress toward goal
- –1 = behavior somewhat worse
- –2 = behavior significantly worse

TABLE 6.5. Steps for Obtaining Goal-Attainment Scaling Ratings

1. Identify independent raters.
2. Gather raters at a single meeting time.
3. Explain that ratings will be done anonymously so that you won't know how any individual rater scored a case (more raters make this easier).
4. Present the range of scores (+2 to –2) and ask raters to consider all the case information before making a judgment and assigning a score.
5. Obtain at least two ratings for each case (on independent score sheets) and take the lower of the two ratings as the score.

This procedure is most efficient and will allow you to get multiple ratings for each case at the same time. Schedule a time for the work and *then* feed them lunch. Third, assure them that their ratings will be anonymous. We suggest that you arrange a pile of cases for them to pick from (taking, for example, from the top and working down).

What kind of information will you need to compile for the raters? At a minimum, you will need a graph of the data (including a goal line that displays the time frame in which the student should have met the goal) and a description of the intervention procedures that were used with the case. If you have any other summary statistics, such as effect sizes or PND, they can be helpful too and should be added to the case file. Case reports that include these items will do nicely.

Fourth, explain to the raters that you want their best judgment according to the criteria in Table 6.4. Finally, we suggest that you arrange for at least two ratings for each case. Two ratings will allow you to examine whether raters tended to agree (were most ratings within ±1 point of each other?). Furthermore, we suggest that you take the *lower* of the two ratings as the actual score. The lower rating is a more conservative (and probably less prone to error) rating of the case. Be sure to make a coding sheet for yourself that identifies the cases for you when the raters are finished. Confidentiality is important. Therefore, assign cases identification numbers that don't mean anything to the raters. The point is to be able to match up the ratings with the cases when the raters are dismissed. *Be very careful to protect client rights to confidentiality by eliminating any information that could potentially identify clients.*

Goal-attainment scaling is the least objective of the measures described in this chapter, so we don't recommend that you rely exclusively on it. However, when it is included as one additional piece of evidence with other evidence such as effect sizes and procedural integrity, it can give an indication of the clinical significance of your outcomes across cases from the perspective of respected but independent colleagues or other stakeholders. It may be the most direct measure of *perceived* clinical significance of your services.

Treatment Integrity

An essential part of evaluating outcomes is determining whether the plan was implemented in the way it was intended in the first place. If the results of an intervention are poor, there are at least two possibilities. Either the intervention was not the right choice for this case or the intervention was not done as planned. This issue is so important that we advise against deciding that a child failed to respond to an intervention until you have firmly documented that the plan was implemented properly and as frequently as intended. In short, the first step in evaluating any intervention is to assess the consistency and frequency with which it was applied—otherwise known as *treatment integrity* or *treatment fidelity*.

Assessing treatment integrity is relatively straightforward if intervention plans are organized as protocols, as are the ones found in Chapters 3, 4, and 5. With such protocols in place, an intervention session can be observed directly by an independent person, who checks whether or not each step was followed. At the end of an intervention session, you can divide the number of steps correctly completed by the total number of steps that were supposed to be followed to determine the percentage of steps correctly completed. If seven steps of an eight-step protocol were followed, the percentage of steps correctly completed is 87.5% for that session. When treatment integrity data are collected for multiple sessions (which is highly advisable), the results can be summarized, like the other data summarization techniques, with descriptive statistics (i.e., mean, median, range, and standard deviation). A high mean and median suggest that the intervention was done mostly correctly (when it *was* done). You can report the percentage of sessions sampled by dividing the number of sessions observed by the total number of intervention sessions administered. For example, if a reading intervention was to be carried out 4 days a week for 8 weeks, there should be 32 intervention sessions in all. If treatment integrity ratings were obtained for 8 sessions, the percentage of sessions sampled was 25%.

Low-treatment integrity can tell you when there is a problem. The person responsible for doing the intervention may not have sufficient knowledge of the procedures. In this case, you will probably need to teach the individual how to do the intervention by coaching and modeling the procedures, observing and prompting the trainee when steps are not followed, and giving feedback (praise for correct implementation and corrective feedback for steps missed or done incorrectly). On the other hand, the person may be knowledgeable but unmotivated. Either the individual doesn't care about changing the situation or other things are competing for his or her time. In some cases, a successful intervention could undermine the objectives of an intervention agent. For example, a teacher who wants a child out of his or her classroom may want to see the intervention fail. (These issues were discussed in greater depth in Chapter 2.) Our point here is to emphasize how you can still take a data-based approach even in this nebulous area of procedural consistency. Summarizing percentage of steps completed over sessions for a particular case gives you some objective numbers to work with when things are not being done so that the issue does not become one of contradictory opinions ("Did too . . . did not . . . did too . . . did not . . .").

There is another positive side to investigating treatment integrity. Good treatment integrity results for a case or a collection of cases suggests that the intervention plans were "doable" (i.e., the persons responsible actually followed through with the procedures in spite of other things that were probably competing for their time) and were probably even acceptable to the person administering them. Why would he or she bother, unless the procedures seemed acceptable and promising? Of course, a person could implement a plan he or she hates. (However, this will be an unlikely explanation in most cases.) Assessing whether the plan was implemented is one part of determining its overall acceptability (Gresham & Lopez, 1996). Gathering systematic treatment integrity data nets one more source of converging evidence about the overall implementation and effectiveness of the intervention plan. Individual case summary statistics (means and medians) can be collated across cases to provide summary statistics (means and medians of individual means and medians) for the program model.

Treatment Acceptability

You can have a case that shows great results on your graph but still be deemed unsuccessful in the eyes of your constituents. If they don't *value* the areas on which you are working or see enough progress, then they probably won't have a very high opinion of the services; for clients and other stakeholders, the treatment and outcomes have low acceptability. Their opinions constitute yet another important source of information for summarizing your overall impact. Of course, from a consultative perspective, you should be working closely with key stakeholders from the very beginning to secure agreement on what you are trying to change and how you will try to elicit that change. Along the way, you should check on acceptability by exploring their preferences, explaining the various ways things can be done and offering choices, and asking for their opinions as unforeseen problems arise. This input is very important information for the case; it is hard, however, to catalogue and organize these unstandardized statements and interactions across cases. The easiest solution is to conduct a survey. If you use a standard survey across cases, you can summarize the results across cases.

There are a number of different acceptability surveys available (Eckert & Hintze, 2000), each with advantages and disadvantages. We have included a simple five-item intervention acceptability survey that has proven very useful in clinical work in Worksheet 6.2. This form can be used flexibly across different types of interventions and can be filled out by teachers, parents, or other key stakeholders. The items are drawn from the Intervention Rating Profile (Martens, Witt, Elliott, & Darveaux, 1985) and represent the five strongest items that assessed overall acceptability. You can give this survey to key stakeholders (e.g., parents) when there are sufficient data to evaluate a treatment plan. Because the items are standard across cases (regardless of the nature of the referral or the intervention), descriptive statistics such as means, medians, range, and standard deviation can be calculated for all cases being reviewed.

Pulling the Data Together and Reporting Results

Now that you know a little something about data summarization methods, you will need to organize your database to facilitate reporting across cases. Like anything else in life, keeping up with this task is half the battle. From a practical standpoint, if you have a plan before you even start taking cases, you can routinely apply certain measures while you are collecting individual case data; doing so will make "pulling it all together" easier in the end. From an evaluation standpoint, it is far better to have a plan for evaluating outcomes before you begin your program than to make it up after the relevant information and data have been collected. We will walk you through the process of planning, maintaining, organizing, and reporting the results (summarized in Table 6.6).

First, you want to start with a database. We recommend creating a file using a spreadsheet program such as Microsoft Excel or an equivalent program. A sample worksheet can be found in Figure 6.3. In this example, there are 13 columns for entering data. The first five columns list relevant identifying information. In most cases, except for the child ID number (which allows you to cancel identifying information, for example, when you have others do goal-attainment scale ratings), this information is confidential and only a limited number of people should be allowed to have access to it. The next two columns identify the "target behavior" (i.e., the area in need of change) and a brief description or name of intervention components. The remaining columns list procedural integrity (i.e., percentage of procedural checklist steps completed), effect sizes, PND, goal-attainment scaling scores, treatment integrity, and acceptability ratings. You will note that there is only one data point in the PND column. In this hypothetical example, PND was calculated only when it was not possible to calculate an effect size. The comprehension intervention for Coughlin presumably had only 2 baseline data points that were equal (e.g., 60% and 60% correct), leaving the standard deviation undefined. Once again, it is not possible to calculate an effect size with an undefined standard deviation. So PND was calculated in this case.

Most of the information can be entered in the database as the cases unfold. For example, as soon as there is a referral, identifying information can be entered. Target behaviors and interventions are identified early in the process and can be entered then. At the end of the intervention period, procedural integrity, effect size, percentage of nonoverlapping data, and treatment integrity can be calculated. Additionally, the Intervention Acceptability Questionnaire (Worksheet 6.2) can be given at this time to parents, teachers, or other key stakeholders. The mean of all five items can serve as the individual case score in the database. Goal-attainment scaling scores can be obtained at one time with a group of raters, as noted above. These data can be entered later, as cases are coming to an end.

Following these steps will allow you to develop a broad, descriptive database such as those reported in the literature for consultative, intervention-based services (e.g., Barnett et al., 1999; Kratochwill et al., 1995). In Figure 6.3, you can see that a range of ages/grades was served across the three primary areas of reading proficiency. A variety of intervention procedures and formats (e.g., peer tutoring, self-monitoring) was used. The quantitative

---

TABLE 6.6. Steps for Collating and Summarizing Data

1. Plan to keep a database and summarize cases as you complete them.

2. Summarize nonquantitative outcomes in terms of
   - Clients served
   - Settings
   - Target behaviors
   - Interventions and their components
   - Intervention agents (who they were)

3. Calculate descriptive statistics (means, medians, range, standard deviation) for each quantitative outcome category and evaluate outcomes.

Child ID	Name	Grade	Sex	Age	Target Behavior(s)	Intervention(s)	Proc. Int.	ES	PND	GAS	TI	Acceptability
0401	Wilkinson	5	F	11	Reading Fluency	RR with peer, self-monitor, reward	100%	2.52		+1	94%	5.4
0402	Stewert	1	M	6	Phon Segmenting	Self-monitoring	87%	1.53		+1	67%	5.6
0403	Newell	2	F	7	Reading Fluency	Peer tutoring (LPP/RR/EC)	92%	1.97		+2	100%	5.2
0404	Michelson	4	M	9	Reading Fluency	Small group (LPP/RR/EC)	100%	058		+1	96%	4.6
0405	Coughlin	6	M	12	Comprehension	Preview questions (RR)	100%		57%	+1	100%	4.8

FIGURE 6.3. A sample database. Proc. Int., procedural integrity; ES, effect size; PND, percentage of nonoverlapping data; GAS, goal-attainment scaling; TI, treatment integrity; Acceptability, mean of five items on the Intervention Acceptability Scale.

data can be summarized as means, medians, ranges, and standard deviations. Most spreadsheet programs will calculate the summary statistics for you. In the example, the mean procedural integrity was 96%, the median was 100%, the standard deviation was 6.02%, and the range was 87–100%. For effect sizes, the mean was 1.65, the median was 1.75, the standard deviation was 0.82, and the range was 0.58–2.52. In the one case where an effect size was not calculable, 57% of the data points was above the highest baseline data point.

For goal-attainment scaling, the mean was 1.2, the median was 1, the standard deviation was 0.45, and the range was 1–2. For treatment integrity, the mean was 91%, the median was 96%, the standard deviation was 13.89%, and the range was 67–100%. For acceptability, the mean was 5.12, the median was 5.2, the standard deviation was 0.41, and the range was 4.2–5.8. Eighty percent of the cases obtained goal-attainment scaling scores of +1, and the remaining case obtained a goal-attainment scaling score of +2. Therefore, the results were uniformly positive for all cases. These data in this hypothetical example would serve as a convincing demonstration of the efficacy of the model, in part, because of the variety of sources of information (adherence to the model, student outcomes, high treatment integrity, and high acceptability) that speak to the overall impact of (1) how well the model was carried out, (2) its effects on students, (3) its effects on those responsible for interventions, and (4) the perceptions of key stakeholders. Since developing it with a colleague a few years ago (see Barnett et al., 1999, for a report of the first year of data), one of us (E.J.D.) has routinely used it when supervising graduate students implementing intervention-based services in schools.

Gauging Your Outcomes: Establishing a Basis for Comparison

We anticipate that some readers will be unfamiliar with at least some of the data synthesis methods just reviewed. When a measure is new to you (e.g., effect sizes), it is hard to gauge exactly what the results mean until you develop a basis for comparison. To that end, Table 6.7 reports the results of a small sample of recent and relevant evaluation studies that use many (and then some) of the measures discussed earlier. Three of the studies are pertinent (Daly & Barnett, 2000; Kratochwill et al., 1995; and McDougal, Clonan, & Martens, 2000) because they report outcomes of intervention-based consultation cases along a number of different dimensions. The first two of these studies (Daly & Barnett, 2000; Kratochwill et al., 1995) document the actual effects of training graduate students in an innovative pilot program of problem-solving intervention-based consultation on real cases. Students were being prepared for these roles, and actual cases provided an opportunity to examine the effectiveness of their training. We found similar, positive outcomes for the training, meaning that even with trainees, the intervention process led to good social consequences for clients in most cases. The McDougal et al. (2000) study examined the same area, but with professionals already working in schools.

The other two studies (Torgesen et al., 2001; Vaughn et al., 2003) report the results of reading interventions that were conducted with groups of students. These studies had more of an instructional focus; they examined various instructional approaches that can be used with students who have reading problems. Nonetheless, you will see that they gathered some of the same types of data to evaluate outcomes. Torgesen et al. (2001) were pri-

TABLE 6.7. Reported Outcomes in the Professional Research Literature (a Sample of Behavioral Consultation and Reading Intervention Evaluation Studies)

Study	Clients	Overall purpose and outcomes

Daly & Barnett (2000)	133 children, ages 3–19 years, preschool through high school (some special education), 67% male, 33% female, 76% white, 20% African American, 4% other	**Purpose**
		Evaluated the outcomes of intervention-based, client-centered services provided by school psychologists in training. Thirty-six consultants in their second year of graduate training provided consultative services for 1 year over a 3-year span on 133 cases in a variety of settings (a Head Start preschool program, public and parochial elementary, middle, and high schools, in both urban and suburban locations). A total of 158 academic and social behaviors were treated through 200 intervention plans that included instructional changes, changes to the classroom environment, reward plans, self-management, classwide interventions, and peer tutoring. Three years of data are reported (the first year is reported by Barnett et al., 1999).
		
		Outcomes
		Procedural checklist (based on a 20-item checklist that described each step that would be followed by the consultant during case management)
		  Year 1: Mean = 97% (SD = 5.4), median = 100%, range = 78–100%
		  Year 2: Mean = 96% (SD = 0.08), median = 100%, range = 60–100%
		  Year 3: Mean = 98% (SD = 3.39), median = 100%, range = 90–100%
		
		Effect sizes
		  Year 1: Mean = 2.86, median = 1.97, range = −.33 to 16.55
		  Year 2: Mean = 1.81, median = 1.25, range = −.99 to 13.1
		  Year 3: Mean = 3.21, median = 1.32, range = −.42 to 49.5
		
		Percentage of nonoverlapping data (PND)
		  Year 1: Mean = 77%, median = 100%, range = 30–100%
		  Year 2: Mean = 76%, median = 100%, range = 0–100%
		  Year 3: Mean = 94%, median = 100%, range = 50–100%
		
		Goal-attainment scaling
		  Year 1: Mean = 1.25 (SD = 0.76), median = 1, range = −1 to +2
		  Year 2: Mean = 1.23 (SD = 0.67), median = 1, range = −1 to +2
		  Year 3: Mean = 1.49 (SD = 0.81), median = 1, range = −1 to +2
		
		Treatment integrity (reported as percentage of steps completed on predetermined intervention plans written in protocol form; each plan was individualized for each case)
		  Year 1: Mean = 86%, median = 97%, range = 0–100%
		  Year 2: Mean = 87%, median = 93%, range = 0–100%
		  Year 3: Mean = 83%, median = 91%, range = 15–100%
		
		Acceptability (on a scale from 1 to 6, with 6 indicating the highest degree of acceptability—"Strongly Agree")
		  Year 1: Mean = 5.37 (SD = 0.61), median = 5, range = 4–6
		  Year 2: Mean = 5.03 (SD = 1.03), median = 5.2, range = 2–6
		  Year 3: Mean = 5.50 (SD = 0.61), median = 5.85, range = 3.9–6

Kratochwill, Elliott, & Busse (1995)	169 children, 3–11 years old, in elementary and preschool grades	**Purpose** Evaluated the effects of training in behavioral consultation for 17 preservice school psychologists over a 5-year period. (Although there was a variety of consultant outcomes, only the degree to which consultants met procedural objectives and client outcomes are reported here.) Consultants were in their first and second year of graduate training. They were grouped by training years (subgroups 1–4). Consultations addressed a variety of behavioral and academic problems. There were whole-classroom interventions, small groups, and individual case consultations.

(continued)

TABLE 6.7. (*continued*)

Study	Clients	Overall purpose and outcomes

Outcomes

Procedural integrity (reported as average percentage of *interview* objectives met by the consultant during actual problem-solving interviews)
    Subgroup 1: 84%; subgroup 2: 90%; subgroup 3: 86%; subgroup 4: 94%

Effect sizes
    Overall mean effect size for 23 cases = .95, range = −.55 to 2.90

Goal-attainment scaling
    Overall mean GAS score = 1.11, median = 1, range = 0 to +2

Acceptability (on a 15-item acceptability survey, with items ranging from 1 to 6, with *6* indicating the highest degree of acceptability; when scores were summed across items, *90* was the highest possible score)
    Overall mean score for 29 cases = 80.3 (*SD* = 6.9)

McDougal, Clonan, & Martens (2000)

47 students in grades K–6 referred for academic and behavioral problems

Purpose

Examined 2 years of outcome data for a school-based intervention team program that was implemented in four urban public elementary schools. Elements of the intervention team process were derived largely from the behavioral consultation literature and implemented in four elementary schools. Careful attention was paid to organizational change processes to increase the chances that the program would become institutionalized in the school district. At the time of the report, the program was in its fourth year.

Outcomes

Procedural integrity (based on 10 objectives of the intervention process that were to be met during multidisciplinary team meetings; ratings were made during unannounced visits by independent observers who rated each objective as either 1 ["met"], 2 ["partially met"], or 3 ["unmet"]; thus, lower ratings are desirable in this case.)
    Overall mean rating for all items = 1.5 (*SD* = 2.9)
    The authors report that "on average . . . the 10 consultative objectives were either met or partially met during 90.5% of observed team meetings" (p. 165).

Acceptability (teacher ratings on a scale from 1 to 6, with *6* being most acceptable; ratings were gathered immediately following team meetings—preintervention—and several weeks after implementing the intervention in the classroom—postintervention.)

	Preint. Mean (*SD*)	Postint. Mean (*SD*)
Comfortable/collaborative atmosphere	5.6 (.83)	—
Helpfulness of intervention team process	5.1 (1.2)	5.1 (1.3)
How the teacher liked the procedures	4.9 (1.1)	4.7 (1.1)
The intervention was a good way to handle the problem	4.7 (.96)	4.6 (1.1)
How beneficial the intervention was for the child	4.7 (1.2)	4.4 (1.6)
There were sufficient resources to implement the intervention	5.0 (.97)	4.8 (1.2)
Overall severity of the problem	5.1 (.91)	4.5 (1.3)

(Follow-up analyses indicate a significant reduction in perceived severity of the problem.)

(*continued*)

TABLE 6.7. *(continued)*

Study	Clients	Overall purpose and outcomes
		Referral rates (comparing referral rates for special education evaluations for the 2 years prior to implementation and the first 2 years of implementation; also, four comparable schools were chosen which were not using the school-based intervention team program.) Year 1: Initial referrals to special education decreased by 22% when compared to the 2 years prior to the project; in contrast, referrals for matched-comparison schools increased by 18%, and overall district referrals increased by 19% during that same year. Year 2: Initial referrals to special education decreased by an additional 15% (yielding an overall reduction of 36% in referrals from preimplementation of the intervention process). Matched schools showed a 3% decrease, whereas the district showed a 4% overall increase in special education referrals.

Torgesen et al. (2001)	60 students with severe reading disabilities between the ages of 8 and 10; participants were classified as learning disabled in the state of Florida	Purpose
		
		The authors delivered two very intense interventions to students to determine whether it would be possible to (1) bring the skills of students with severe reading disabilities to average levels of performance, (2) determine whether there were significant differences between treatments, and (3) examine whether either method would be differentially effective for children with different cognitive, linguistic, and demographic profiles. Outcomes were measured in the areas of phonemic decoding, word identification, and passage comprehension. (Refer to the original study for a detailed description of outcomes in each of these areas. Only effect sizes and outcomes relative to continuation in special education placement are reported here.) Students received 67.5 hours of one-on-one instruction in two 50-minute sessions per day for 8 weeks in either an Auditory Discrimination in Depth program or an Embedded Phonics program.
		
		Outcomes
		
		Effect sizes (comparing growth during intervention to the participants' growth during the previous 16 months in learning disabilities resource rooms)
		    Auditory Discrimination in Depth: 4.4
		    Embedded Phonics: 3.9
		
		Exited from special education
		The authors report that "approximately 40% of the children were judged to be no longer in need of special education services and were returned full-time to the general education classroom within the first year following the end of the intervention" (p. 50).

(continued)

TABLE 6.7. (*continued*)

Study	Clients	Overall purpose and outcomes
Vaughn, Linan-Thompson, & Hickman (2003)	45 second-grade students at risk for reading problems who were not already receiving supplemental reading instruction and who had failed the second-grade Texas Primary Reading Inventory screening; 35 students were Hispanic, 6 were white, and 4 were African American	

Purpose

This study was intended to examine (1) the number of students who would meet predetermined exit criteria, following daily supplemental reading instruction; (2) the degree to which students who improved during supplemental instruction and met exit criteria would be successful in general education when supplemental instruction was terminated; and (3) "the feasibility of using a response-to-treatment model to identify students with LD by a school or district" (p. 384). Exit criteria included (1) a passing score on the Texas Primary Reading Inventory: Screening (i.e., five or more words, out of eight, read correctly), (2) reading at least 55 correct read words per minute on a second-grade-level passage of the Test of Oral Reading Fluency, and (3) reading at least 50 correct read words per minute, for at least 3 consecutive weeks, in second-grade fluency progress-monitoring sessions. Supplemental instruction focused on phonemic awareness, phonics (especially sound–letter relationships and word families), word and text reading fluency, instructional level reading and comprehension, and spelling; delivered daily for 35 minutes in small groups. Four tutors provided supplemental instruction.

Outcomes

Outcomes are reported by students' category of when they met exit criteria: after 10 weeks, 20 weeks, 30 weeks, or never.

Number of students who met exit criteria at different intervals

Met after 10 weeks:	10
Met after 20 weeks:	14
Met after 30 weeks:	10
Never met exit criteria:	11

Effect sizes	During intervention	At 30-week follow-up
Met after 10 weeks:	2.74	1.72
Met after 20 weeks:	3.23	0.97
Met after 30 weeks:	6.06	6.06
Never met exit criteria:	2.66	2.66

Intervention validity checklist (a treatment integrity checklist on which features of instruction were recorded; quality of instruction was judged by independent observers for activities and materials as well as instructional time on a scale from 0 (not observed) to 3 (observed most of the time); results are reported for each area of instruction.)

Fluency: Mean rating = 2.53 (*SD* = 0.15), median = 2.5
Phonological awareness: Mean rating = 2.5 (*SD* = 0.39), median = 2.55
Instructional reading: Mean rating = 2.6 (*SD* = 0.48), median = 2.8
Word analysis: Mean rating = 2.55 (*SD* = 0.37), median = 2.5

marily interested in effects that could be achieved with a very strong and intense intervention. From the perspective of the children served, their efforts certainly "paid off." The Vaughn et al. (2003) study is unique because it operationalized reading problems from a response-to-intervention perspective (discussed earlier in this chapter). The study should allow schools to estimate the degree of success they might expect within and across students if they use a similar model for identifying and treating reading problems *before* classifying the students as learning disabled.

Not all of the data have been reported for each of the studies. Only data germane to our purposes are used to illustrate how some of these different data analysis methods of reporting results to others might be summarized. How will your data compare with the data reported in these studies? You can use the findings from these studies as a benchmark for gauging your success. There are two outcomes reported in these studies that are not discussed above but which might be an important source of information to you. For example, McDougal et al. (2000) synthesized building and district referral rates for special education evaluations. Their data suggest that (1) there were clear reductions in the number of referrals to special education in buildings where school-based intervention teams (SBIT) operated, (2) referrals remained stable in comparable school buildings without the SBIT process, and (3) referrals districtwide increased. Torgesen et al. (2001) tackled severe reading problems and were able to report an amazing percentage of students who were discharged from special education classes. This type of information is very persuasive with other professionals and constituents because it contains the types of data that school districts are routinely gathering in the first place. They just need to be "mined" by people who have the vision to ascertain how their reading intervention program compares to similar programs in other schools, and how their program affects the educational placements of participating students. Each of these reports contains an impressive amount of information, and we advise the interested reader to obtain the original publications. They are a good read—and they will help you to further refine your evaluation plan.

Sharing Your Results with Others

Sharing your results may be as important a task as all your intervention and data collection efforts, if continuation of your program or funding for your program hinges on convincing others of its positive impact on students. Whether it be through a written report or an oral presentation to a group, you want to have a crisp, clear, and professional format for presenting your results—and then you can let the data speak for "themselves." Graphs efficiently display a lot of information and require only simple explanations for people to grasp what they mean. They are also satisfying for consumers once they understand what the results mean, because then they can judge for themselves whether or not the results are convincing.

We strongly encourage you to create one or more graphs of quantitative outcomes in any reporting you do. You will find sample graphs in Figures 6.4 and 6.5. Effect sizes, goal-attainment scaling, and intervention acceptability means are displayed in a bar-graph format, using data reported by Daly and Barnett (2000). Three years of data are reported in each graph. As noted previously, you can create the same reporting format over time by

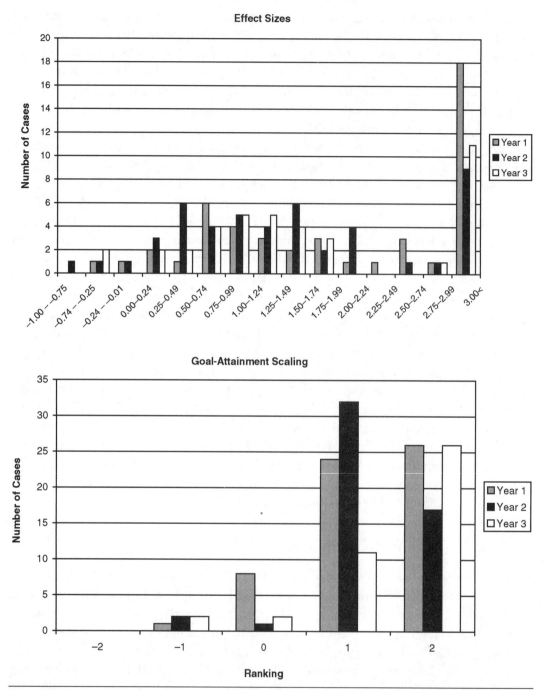

FIGURE 6.4. Summary graphs of effect sizes and goal-attainment scaling. From Daly and Barnett (2000). Reprinted by permission of the authors.

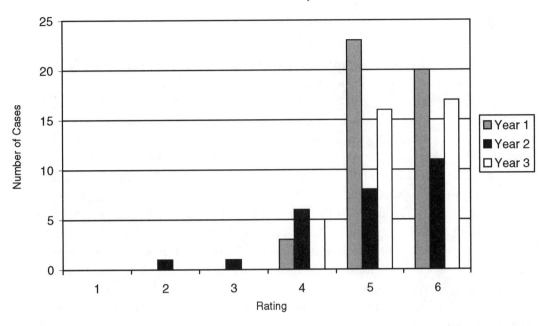

FIGURE 6.5. Summary graph of intervention acceptability data. From Daly and Barnett (2000). Reprinted by permission of the authors.

using simple charting tools contained in spreadsheet programs such as Microsoft Excel® or the "Chart Dog" feature at *interventioncentral.org*. Such graphs allow reviewers to see the range of outcomes obtained, where the results cluster, and, when there are data for multiple years, whether the results are consistent over time.

Tables may be helpful for displaying more descriptive statistics than just the mean. For instance, Table 6.8 contains information on number of cases per year, means, medians, and range of procedural checklist outcomes (reported as a percentage of steps completed; data from Daly and Barnett, 2000). Once again, data displays such as this one are packed with useful information. As the presenter, you can draw the attention of those reviewing the data to different features in the results, such as overall patterns, how much variability there is in the results, and whether there were changes over years or according to types of cases (if you break down the data in this way). It is helpful to try plotting your data in various ways to determine which method (1) communicates the most information and (2) highlights the key findings.

TABLE 6.8. Procedural Checklist Outcomes

Year	No. reported	Mean (*SD*)	Median	Range
1	70	97% (5.4)	100	78–100%
2	36	96% (0.08)	100	60–100%
3	37	98% (3.39)	100	90–100%

Note. From Daly and Barnett (2000). Reprinted by permission of the authors.

CONCLUSION

Whereas the other chapters in this book gave you the tools to understand your consultative task in the broader context of classroom and school needs (Chapters 1 and 2) and how to conduct your services (Chapters 3, 4, and 5), this chapter has emphasized a rationale and techniques for how to conceptualize and analyze the outcomes of those services. Each part of the model presented in this book prepares you for the next step in the process. In some ways, though, the consultation process is like a juggling act. You have to keep several pieces going at once: staying informed about organizational priorities in schools where you are working, being knowledgeable about interventions, and planning overall evaluation to justify your services. Evaluation is the key to it all, whether it is evaluation of the individual child or of an entire program. Evaluation should drive the whole process—staying on course, as originally planned, or making changes. Evaluation is a purposeful, planned, and ongoing activity. All procedures of the process (except the activity of evaluation itself) should be subject to revision contingent on evaluation results. This principle applies to the repeated readings intervention being used with a third-grade student who is behind in reading as well as to the procedures followed for each case by a multidisciplinary prereferral intervention team. This whole discussion implies, however, that you have an evaluation plan that is sensitive to detecting meaningful changes over time. This is where antiquated methods of identifying reading disabilities displayed their flaws. The IQ–achievement discrepancy approach landed students in special education classes, but it didn't provide information useful to their programming and could not tell us whether they were actually getting better. A sense of complacency may be what led educators to live with these circumstances for so long, before the winds of accountability and change started stirring up the sand. Now is the time to act with a purpose and an end in sight! You have the means to discover whether you are getting there.

WORKSHEET 6.1. Procedural Checklist

Procedural steps   **Date completed**

1. Obtain parent permission and discuss the problem and available
   resources with parent, teacher(s), and other stakeholders (SPECIFY:
   _____)   _____

2. Establish a baseline (minimum of 3 data points with standardized
   procedures for assessing early literacy, reading fluency, and/or
   reading comprehension) and display the results on a graph.   _____

3. Establish a data-based goal that describes the learner, conditions of
   ongoing assessment (time and materials for responding), how many
   corrects and incorrects are expected (expected performance), and a
   goal date. Draw the goal on the graph.   _____

4. An intervention plan is established that describes what will be done,
   where, when, how many times a week, how long (per session), by
   whom, and with what resources. The plan is written out and shared
   with the parents and other team members.   _____

5. A plan evaluation date and time are set for no more than 8 weeks
   after the first plan is established. (SPECIFY DATE AND TIME:
   _____)   _____

6. Arrangements are made for an independent person to directly
   observe whether the plan is being done during scheduled sessions. A
   recording plan is established for determining how many steps were
   correctly followed during scheduled intervention sessions.   _____

7. At least 8–10 data points are gathered during the intervention period.
   (SPECIFY BY WHOM: _____)   _____

8. The plan is evaluated according to: _____
   (a) whether the plan was carried out as intended and as frequently
       as intended; and
   (b) whether the student is progressing toward meeting the goal.

9. Agreement is achieved on the decision to: _____
   • Continue the plan unmodified.
   • Modify the plan.
   • Terminate the plan.
       (Check the appropriate box and explain the decision and next
   steps at the end of the checklist.)

10. The acceptability of the plan, process, and results were assessed with
    the acceptability questionnaire by the parent, the child, and the
    teacher.   _____

WORKSHEET 6.2. Intervention Acceptability Scale

Child's Name: _____

Name of rater and relationship with child: _____

Date: _____

Intervention: _____

Please rate the intervention procedures using the following scale:

    1 = Strongly Disagree
    2 = Disagree
    3 = Slightly Disagree
    4 = Slightly Agree
    5 = Agree
    6 = Strongly Agree

1.	I like the procedures used in this intervention.	1	2	3	4	5	6
2.	This intervention is a good way to handle this problem.	1	2	3	4	5	6
3.	Overall, this intervention is beneficial for the student.	1	2	3	4	5	6
4.	This intervention is reasonable for the problem.	1	2	3	4	5	6
5.	I would be willing to use this intervention in the classroom setting in the future.	1	2	3	4	5	6

Please make any comments below. Use the back if necessary.

References

Adams, M. J. (1990). *Beginning to read: Thinking and learning about print*. Cambridge, MA: MIT Press.

Adams, M. J., Foorman, B., Lundberg, I., & Beeler, T. (1998). *Phonemic awareness in young children*. Baltimore: Brookes.

Adelman, H. S. (1982). Identifying learning problems at an early age: A critical appraisal. *Journal of Clinical Child Psychology, 11*, 255–261.

Alesandri, K. L. (1982). Imagery-eliciting strategy and meaningful learning. *Journal of Mental Imagery, 6*, 125–141.

American Psychological Association. (2001). *Publication manual of the American Psychological Association* (5th ed.). Washington, DC: Author.

Anderman, R. C., & Williams, J. M. (1986, April). *Teaching test-taking and note-taking skills to learning disabled high school students*. Paper presented at the Annual Convention of the Council for Exceptional Children, New Orleans, LA (ERIC Document Reproduction Service No. ED268772).

Ball, E. W., & Blachman, B. A. (1991). Does phoneme awareness training in kindergarten make a difference in early word recognition and developmental spelling? *Reading Research Quarterly, 26*, 49–66.

Barnett, D. W., Daly, E. J., III, Hampshire, E. M., Hines, N. R., Maples, K. A., Ostrom, J. K., & Van Buren, A. E. (1999). Meeting performance-based training demands: Accountability in an intervention-based practicum. *School Psychology Quarterly, 14*, 357–379.

Barnett, D. W., Lentz, F. E., Jr., & Macmann, G. (2000). Psychometric qualities of professional practice. In E. S. Shapiro & T. R. Kratochwill (Eds.), *Behavioral assessment in schools: Theory, research, and clinical foundations* (2nd ed., pp. 355–386). New York: Guilford Press.

Barnett, D. W., & Macmann, G. M. (1992). Aptitude–achievement discrepancy scores: Accuracy in analysis misdirected. *School Psychology Review, 21*, 494–508.

Beck, I. L. (1997, October/November). Response to "overselling phonics." *Reading Today*, p. 17.

Blachman, B. A. (1994). Early literacy acquisition: The role of phonological awareness. In G. P. Wallach & K. G. Butler (Eds.), *Language learning disabilities in school-aged children and adolescents* (pp. 253–274). New York: Merrill.

Blachman, B. A., Ball, E. W., Black, R. S., & Tangel, D. M. (2000). *Road to the code: A phonological awareness program for young children.* Baltimore: Brookes.

Blum, I. H., & Koskinen, P. S. (1991). Prompted reading: A strategy for enhancing fluency and fostering expertise. *Theory into Practice, 30,* 195–200.

Bos, C. S., & Anders, P. L. (1990). Interactive practice for teaching content and strategic knowledge. In T. E. Scruggs & B. Y. L. Wong (Eds.), *Intervention research in learning disabilities* (pp. 116–185). New York: Springer-Verlag.

Bos, C. S., Anders, P. L., Filip, D., & Jaffe, L. E. (1989). The effects of an interactive instructional strategy for enhancing reading comprehension and content area learning for students with learning disabilities. *Journal of Learning Disabilities, 22,* 384–390.

Boyle, J. R., Weishaar, M. (2001). The effects of strategic notetaking on the recall and comprehension of lecture information for high school students with learning disabilities. *Learning Disabilities Research and Practice, 16,* 133–141.

Brandoof-Matter, E. (1989). Visualize to improve comprehension. *Reading Teacher, 42,* 338.

Busk, P. L., & Serlin, R. C. (1992). Meta-analysis for single-case research. In T. R. Kratochwill & J. R. Levin (Eds.), *Single-case research design and analysis: Applications in psychology and education* (pp. 187–212). Hillsdale, NJ: Erlbaum.

Carnine, D. W. (1976). Effects of two teacher presentation rates of off-task behavior, answering correctly, and participation. *Journal of Applied Behavior Analysis, 9,* 199–206.

Carnine, D., & Kinder, B. D. (1985). Teaching low-performing students to apply generative and schema strategies to narrative and expository material. *Remedial and Special Education, 6,* 20–30.

Catts, H. W. (1995). *Language basics of reading disabilities: Implications for early identification and remediation.* Paper presented at the annual conference of the Speech, Language, and Hearing Association of Alberta, Canada.

Chafouleas, S. M., Lewandowski, L. J., Smith, C. R., & Blachman, B. A. (1997). Phonological awareness skills in children: Examining performance across tasks and ages. *Journal of Psychoeducational Assessment, 15,* 334–347.

Chafouleas, S. M., VanAuken, T., & Dunham, K. (2001). Not all phonemes are created equal: The effects of linguistic manipulations on phonological awareness tasks. *Journal of Psychoeducational Assessment, 19,* 216–226.

Chan, L. K. S., Cole, P. G., & Barfett, S. (1987). Comprehension monitoring: Detection and identification of text inconsistencies by learning disabled and normal students. *Learning Disability Quarterly, 10,* 144–124.

Chan, L. K. S., Cole, P. G., & Morris, J. N. (1990). Effect of instruction in the use of visual-imagery strategy on the reading-comprehension competence of disabled and average readers. *Learning Disability Quarterly, 13,* 1–11.

Chard, D. J., Vaughn, S., & Tyler, B. J. (2002). A synthesis of research on effective interventions for building reading fluency with elementary students with learning disabilities. *Journal of Learning Disabilities, 35,* 386–406.

Chomsky, C. (1978). When you still can't read in third grade: After decoding, what? In S. J. Samuels (Ed.), *What research has to say about reading instruction* (pp. 13–30). Newark, DE: International Reading Association.

Cohen, J. (1988). *Statistical power analysis for the behavioral sciences.* Hillsdale, NJ: Erlbaum.

Cone, J. D. (2001). *Evaluating outcomes: Empirical tools for effective practice.* Washington, DC: American Psychological Association.

Cunningham, J. W. (1979). An automatic pilot for decoding. *Reading Teacher, 32,* 420–424.

D'Alessio, J. A. (1996). *Retelling in the improvement of reading comprehension scores of urban, lower socio-economic fourth graders.* MA project, Kean College of New Jersey, Union, NJ (ERIC Document Reproduction No. ED 394135).

Daly, E. J., III, & Barnett, D. W. (2000). *Meeting performance-based demands for practicum training: Three years of data.* Paper presented at the annual convention of the National Association of School Psychologists, New Orleans.

Daly, E. J., III, Chafouleas, S. M., Persampieri, M., Bonfiglio, C. M., & Lafleur, K. (2004). Teaching phoneme segmenting and blending as critical early literacy skills: An experimental analysis of minimal textual repertoires. *Journal of Behavioral Education, 13,* 165–178.

Daly, E. J., III, Garbacz, S. A., Olson, S. C., Persampieri, M., & Ni, H. (in press). Improving oral reading fluency by influencing students' choice of instructional procedures: An experimental analysis with two students with behavioral disorders. *Behavioral Interventions.*

Daly, E. J., III, Hintze, J. M., & Hamler, K. R. (2000). Improving practice by taking steps toward technological improvements in academic intervention in the new millennium. *Psychology in the Schools, 37,* 61–72.

Daly, E. J., III, Lentz, F. E., & Boyer, J. (1996). The instructional hierarchy: A conceptual model for understanding the effective components of reading interventions. *School Psychology Quarterly, 11,* 369–386.

Daly, E. J., III, & Martens, B. K. (1994). A comparison of three interventions for increasing oral reading performance: Application of the instructional hierarchy. *Journal of Applied Behavior Analysis, 27,* 459–469.

Daly, E. J., III, Martens, B. K., Dool, E. J., & Hintze, J. M. (1998). Using brief functional analysis to select interventions for oral reading. *Journal of Behavioral Education, 8,* 203–218.

Daly, E. J., III, Martens, B. K., Kilmer, A., & Massie, D. (1996). The effects of instructional match and content overlap on generalized reading performance. *Journal of Applied Behavior Analysis, 29,* 507–518.

Daly, E. J., III, & Murdoch, A. (2000). Direct observation in the assessment of academic skill problems. In E. S. Shapiro & T. R. Kratochwill (Eds.), *Behavioral assessment in schools: Theory, research, and clinical foundations* (2nd ed., pp. 46–77). New York: Guilford Press.

Daly, E. J., III, Wright, J. A., Kelly, S. Q., & Martens, B. K. (1997). Measures of early academic skills: Reliability and validity with a first-grade sample. *School Psychology Quarterly, 12,* 268–280.

Daneman, M., & Carpenter, P. A. (1980). Individual differences in working memory and reading. *Journal of Verbal Learning and Behavior, 19,* 450–466.

Dawes, R. M. (1994). *House of cards: Psychology and psychotherapy built on myth.* New York: Free Press.

Dawes, R. M. (1995). Standards of practice. In S. C. Hayes, V. M. Follette, R. M. Dawes, & K. E. Grady (Eds.), *Scientific standards of psychological practice: Issues and recommendations* (pp. 49–66). Reno, NV: Context Press.

Deno, S. L., Fuchs, L. S., Marston, D., & Shin, J. (2001). Using curriculum-based measurement to establish growth standards for students with learning disabilities. *School Psychology Review, 30,* 507–524.

Dowhower, S. L. (1987). Effects of repeated reading on second-grade transitional readers' fluency and comprehension. *Reading Research Quarterly, 22,* 389–406.

Duke, N. K., & Pearson, P. D. (2002). Effective practices for developing reading comprehension. In A. E. Farstrup & S. J. Samuels (Eds.), *What research has to say about reading instruction* (pp. 205–242). Newark, DE: International Reading Association.

Eckert, T. L., Ardoin, S. P., Daly, E. J., III, & Martens, B. K. (2002). Improving oral reading fluency:

An examination of the efficacy of combining skill-based and performance-based interventions. *Journal of Applied Behavior Analysis, 35,* 271–281.

Eckert, T. L., & Hintze, J. M. (2000). Behavioral conceptions and applications of acceptability: Issues related to service delivery and research methodology. *School Psychology Quarterly, 15,* 123–148.

Englemann, S., Granzin, A., & Severson, H. (1979). Diagnosing instruction. *Journal of Special Education, 13,* 355–363.

Englert, C. S., & Mariage, T. V. (1991). Making students partners in the comprehension process: Organizing the reading "POSSE." *Learning Disability Quarterly, 14,* 123–138.

Erchul, W. P., & Martens, B. K (2002). *School consultation: Conceptual and empirical bases of practice* (2nd ed.). New York: Plenum Press.

Fahmy, J. J., & Bilton, L. (1990, April). *Lecture comprehension and note-taking for L2 students.* Paper presented at the World Congress of Applied Linguistics, Thessalonica, Greece (ERIC Document Reproduction Service No. ED323785).

Fox, B., & Routh, D. K. (1975). Analyzing spoken language into words, syllables, and phonemes: A developmental study. *Journal of Psycholinguistic Research, 4,* 331–342.

Freeland, J. T., Skinner, C. H., Jackson, B., McDaniel, C. E., & Smith, S. (2000). Measuring and increasing silent reading comprehension rates via repeated readings. *Psychology in the Schools, 37,* 415–429.

Freeman, T. J., & McLaughlin, T. F. (1984). Effects of a taped-words treatment procedure on learning disabled students' sight-word reading. *Learning Disability Quarterly, 7,* 49–54.

Fuchs, L. S., & Deno, S. L. (1982). *Developing goals and objectives for educational programs* (Teaching guide). Minneapolis: Institute for Research in Learning Disabilities, University of Minnesota.

Fuchs, L. S., & Deno, S. L. (1994). Must instructionally useful performance assessment be based in the curriculum? *Exceptional Children, 57,* 488–500.

Fuchs, L. S., & Fuchs, D. (1998). Treatment validity: A unifying concept for reconceptualizing the identification of learning disabilities. *Learning Disabilities Research and Practice, 13,* 204–219.

Fuchs, L. S., & Fuchs, D. (1999). Monitoring student progress toward the development of reading competence: A review of three forms of classroom-based assessment. *School Psychology Review, 28,* 659–671.

Fuchs, L. S., Fuchs, D., Hamlett, C. L., Walz, L., & Germann, G. (1993). Formative evaluation of academic progress: How much growth can we expect? *School Psychology Review, 22,* 27–48.

Fuchs, L. S., Fuchs, D., Hosp, M. K., & Jenkins, J. R. (2001). Oral reading fluency as an indicator of reading competence: A theoretical, empirical, and historical analysis. *Scientific Studies of Reading, 5,* 239–256.

Fuchs, L. S., Fuchs, D., & Speece, D. L. (2002). Treatment validity as a unifying construct for identifying learning disabilities. *Learning Disabilities Quarterly, 25,* 33–45.

Gaskins, I. W., Ehri, L. C., & Cress, C. (1996). Procedures for word learning: Making discoveries about words—Benchmark Word Identification program. *Reading Teacher, 50,* 312–327.

Gettinger, M. (1995). Increasing academic learning time. In A. Thomas & J. Grimes (Eds.), *Best practices in school psychology III* (pp. 943–954). Washington, DC: National Association of School Psychologists.

Gickling, E. E., & Rosenfield, S. (1995). Best practices in curriculum-based assessment. In A. Thomas & J. Grimes (Eds.), *Best practices in school psychology III* (pp. 587–596). Washington, DC: National Association of School Psychologists.

Giesen, C., & Peeck, J. (1984). The effect of imagery instruction on reading and retaining of literary text. *Journal of Mental Imagery, 8*(2), 79–90.

Good, R. H., & Kaminski, R. A. (Eds.). (2001). *Dynamic indicators of basic early literacy skills.* Eugene, OR: Institute for the Development of Educational Achievement. (Available online at *http://dibels.uoregon.edu/*)

Good, R. H., Kaminski, R. A., & Smith, S. (2002). Word use fluency. In R. H. Good & R. A. Kaminski (Eds.), *Dynamic indicators of basic early literacy skills* (6th ed.). Eugene, OR: Institute for the Development of Educational Achievement. (Available online at *http://dibels.uoregon.edu/*)

Good, R. H., III, & Shinn, M. R. (1990). Forecasting accuracy of slope estimates for reading curriculum-based measurement: Empirical evidence. *Behavioral Assessment, 12,* 179–193.

Graham, L., & Wong, B. Y. L. (1993). Comparing two modes of teaching a question-answering strategy for enhancing reading comprehension: Didactic and self-instructional training. *Journal of Learning Disabilities, 26,* 270–279.

Granowsky, A. (2000). Dinosaur fossils. *Open Court Reading Book 1 Grade 2.* Columbus, OH: McGraw-Hill.

Gravois, T. A., & Gickling, E. E. (2002). Best practices in curriculum-based assessment. In A. Thomas & J. Grimes (Eds.), *Best practices in school psychology* (4th ed., pp. 885–898). Bethesda, MD: National Association of School Psychologists.

Greenwood, C. R. (1991a). Classwide peer tutoring: Longitudinal effects on the reading, language, and mathematics achievement of at-risk students. *Reading, Writing, and Learning Disabilities, 7,* 105–123.

Greenwood, C. R. (1991b). Longitudinal analysis of time, engagement, and achievement in at-risk versus non-risk students. *Exceptional Children, 57,* 521–535.

Greenwood, C. R., Delquadri, J. C., & Carta, J. J. (1997). *Together we can!: Classwide peer tutoring to improve basic academic skills.* Longmont, CO: Sopris West.

Greenwood, C. R., Delquadri, J., & Hall, R. V. (1984). Opportunity to respond and student academic performance. In W. L. Heward, T. E. Heron, J. Trap-Porter, & D. S. Hill (Eds.), *Focus on behavior analysis in education* (pp. 58–88). Columbus, OH: Merrill.

Greenwood, C. R., Delquadri, J., & Hall, R. V. (1989). Longitudinal effects of classwide peer tutoring. *Journal of Educational Psychology, 81,* 371–383.

Greenwood, C. R., Terry, B., Marquis, J., & Walker, D. (1994). Confirming a performance-based instructional model. *School Psychology Review, 23,* 652–668.

Gresham, F. M. (2001). *Responsiveness to intervention: An alternative approach to the identification of learning disabilities.* Paper prepared for the OSEP Learning Disabilities Initiative, Office of Special Education Program, U.S. Department of Education, Washington, DC.

Gresham, F. M., & Lopez, M. F. (1996). Social validation: A unifying concept for school-based consultation research and practice. *School Psychology Quarterly, 11,* 204–227.

Grossen, B., & Carnine, D. (1991). Strategies for maximizing reading success in the regular classroom. In G. Stoner, M. R. Shinn, & H. M. Walker (Eds.), *Interventions for achievement and behavior problems* (pp. 333–356). Bethesda, MD: National Association of School Psychologists.

Gunn, B. K., Simmons, D. C., & Kame'enui, E. J. (1995). *Emergent literacy: Synthesis of the research.* (Available online at *http://idea.uoregon.edu/~ncite/documents/techrep/tech19.html*)

Hargis, C. H. (1995). *Curriculum-based assessment: A primer* (2nd ed.). Springfield, IL: Thomas.

Haring, N. G., Lovitt, T. C., Eaton, M. D., & Hansen, C. L. (1978). *The fourth R: Research in the classroom*. Columbus, OH: Merrill.

Harper, G. L., Maheady, L., Mallette, B., & Karnes, M. (1999). Peer tutoring and the minority child with disabilities. *Preventing School Failure, 43*, 45–51.

Hasbrouck, J. E., & Tindal, G. (1992). Curriculum-based oral reading fluency norms for students in grades 2 through 5. *Teaching Exceptional Children, 24*, 41–44.

Hintze, J. M, Callahan, J. E., III, Matthews, W. J., Williams, S. A. S., & Tobin, K. G. (2002). Oral reading fluency and prediction of reading comprehension in African American and Caucasian elementary school children. *School Psychology Review, 31*, 540–553.

Horner, R. D., & Baer, D. M. (1978). Multiple-probe technique: A variation of the multiple baseline design. *Journal of Applied Behavior Analysis, 11*, 189–196.

Hoskisson, K., & Krohm, B. (1974). Reading by immersion: Assisted reading. *Elementary English, 51*, 832–836.

Howell, K. W., & Kelly, B. (2002). Curriculum clarification, lesson design, and delivery. In K. L. Lane, F. M. Gresham, & T. E. O'Shaughnessy (Eds.), *Interventions for children with or at risk for emotional and behavioral disorders* (pp. 57–73). Boston: Allyn & Bacon.

Howell, K. W., & Nolet, V. (2000). *Curriculum-based evaluation: Teaching and decision making* (3rd ed.). Belmont, CA: Wadsworth.

Idol-Maestas, L. (1985). Getting ready to read: Guided probing for poor comprehenders. *Learning Disability Quarterly, 8*, 243–254.

Jackson, B. J., Freeland, J. T., & Skinner, C. H. (2000, November). *Using reading previewing to improve reading comprehension rates for secondary student with reading deficits*. Paper presented at the annual meeting of the Mid-South Educational Research Association, Bowling Green, KY.

Jacob, S., & Hartshorne, T. (2003). *Ethics and law for school psychologists* (4th ed.). New York: Wiley.

Jones, K. M., & Wickstrom, K. F. (2002). Done in sixty seconds: Further analysis of the brief assessment model for academic problems. *School Psychology Review, 31*, 554–568.

Kame'enui, E. J., & Simmons, D. C. (2001). Introduction to this special issue: The DNA of reading fluency. *Scientific Studies of Reading, 5*, 203–210.

Kaminiski, R. A., & Good, R. H. (1996). Toward a technology for assessing basic early literacy skills. *School Psychology Review, 25*, 215–227.

Kamps, D. M., Barbetta, P. M., Leonard, B. R., & Delquadri, J. (1994). Classwide peer tutoring: An integration strategy to improve reading skills and promote peer interactions among students with autism and general education peers. *Journal of Applied Behavior Analysis, 27*, 49–61.

Kavale, A. K., & Forness, S. R. (1999). Effectiveness of special education. In C. R. Reynolds & T. B. Gutkin (Eds.), *The handbook of school psychology* (3rd ed., pp. 984–1024). New York: Wiley.

Kinder, D., & Carnine, D. (1991). Direct instruction: What it is and what it is becoming. *Journal of Behavioral Education, 1*, 193–213.

Koltun, H., & Biemiller, A. (1999, April). *Metacognition of vocabulary knowledge: A preliminary study*. Paper presented at the annual meeting of the American Educational Research Association, Montreal, Quebec, Canada (ERIC Document Reproduction Service No. ED433350).

Kranzler, J. H., Brownell, M. T., & Miller, M. D. (1998). The construct validity of curriculum-based measurement of reading: An empirical test of a plausible rival hypothesis. *Journal of School Psychology, 36*, 399–415.

Kratochwill, T. R., Elliott, S. N., & Busse, R. T. (1995). Behavior consultation: A five-year evaluation of consultant and client outcomes. *School Psychology Quarterly, 10*, 87–117.

LaBerge, D., & Samuels, S. J. (1974). Toward a theory of automatic information processing in reading. *Cognitive Psychology, 6*, 293–323.

Lane, K. L., Gresham, F. M., & O'Shaughnessy, T. E. (Eds.). (2002). *Interventions for children with or at risk for emotional and behavioral disorders*. Boston: Allyn & Bacon.

Leal, D. (1993). The power of literacy peer-group discussions: How children collaboratively negotiate meaning. *Reading Teacher, 47*, 114–121.

Lentz, F. E., Allen, S. J., & Ehrhardt, K. E. (1996). The conceptual elements of strong interventions in school settings. *School Psychology Quarterly, 11*, 118–136.

Lesgold, A. M., & Perfetti, C. A. (1978). Interactive processes in reading comprehension. *Discourse Processes, 1*, 323–336.

Lesgold, A. M., & Resnick, L. (1982). How reading difficulties develop: Perspectives from a longitudinal study. In J. Das, R. Mulcahy, & A. Wall (Eds.), *Theory and research in learning disabilities* (pp. 155–187). New York: Plenum Press.

Liberman, I. Y., Shankweiler, D., Fischer, F. W., & Carter, B. (1974). Explicit syllable and phoneme segmentation in the young child. *Journal of Experimental Child Psychology, 18*, 201–212.

Lindamood, P., & Lindamood, P. (1998). *The Lindamood phoneme sequencing program for reading, spelling, and speech*. Austin, TX: PRO-ED.

Lloyd, C. V. (1995–1996). How teachers teach reading comprehension: An examination of four categories of reading comprehension instruction. *Reading Research and Instruction, 35*, 171–185.

Lovitt, T., Rudest, J., Jenkins, J., Pious, C., & Benedetti, D. (1986). Adapting science materials for regular and learning disabled seventh graders. *Remedial and Special Education, 7*(1), 31–39.

Mace, F. C., McCurdy, B., & Quigley, E. A. (1990). The collateral effect of reward predicted by matching theory. *Journal of Applied Behavior Analysis, 23*, 197–205.

Mace, F. C., Neef, N. A., Shade, D., & Mauro, B. C. (1996). Effects of problem difficulty and reinforcer quality on time allocated to concurrent arithmetic problems. *Journal of Applied Behavior Analysis, 29*, 11–24.

Macmann, G. M., & Barnett, D. W. (1999). Diagnostic decision making in school psychology: Understanding and coping with uncertainty. In C. R. Reynolds & T. Gutkin (Eds.), *The handbook of school psychology* (3rd ed., pp. 519–548). New York: Wiley.

Macon, L. (Ed.). (1991). *Learning disabilities in the high school: A methods booklet for secondary special subject teachers*. Pittsburgh, PA: Learning Disabilities Association of America.

MacQuarrie, L. L., Tucker, J. A., Burns, M. K., & Hartman, B. (2002). Comparison of retention rates using traditional, drill sandwich, and incremental rehearsal flash card methods. *School Psychology Review, 31*, 584–595.

Marston, D. B. (1989). A curriculum-based measurement approach to assessing academic performance: What it is and when to do it. In M. R. Shinn (Ed.), *Curriculum-based measurement: Assessing special children* (pp. 18–78). New York: Guilford Press.

Marston, D. B., & Magnusson, D. (1988). Curriculum-based measurement: District-level implementation. In J. L. Graden, J. E. Zins, & M. J. Curtis (Eds.), *Alternative educational delivery systems: Enhancing options for all students* (pp. 137–172). Washington, DC: National Association of School Psychologists.

Marston, D., & Tindal, G. (1995). Performance monitoring. In A. Thomas & J. Grimes (Eds.), *Best practices in school psychology III* (pp. 597–608). Washington, DC: National Association of School Psychologists.

Martens, B. K., Witt, J. C., Elliott, S. N., & Darveaux, D. (1985). Teacher judgments concerning the acceptability of school-based interventions. *Professional Psychology: Research and Practice, 16*, 191–198.

McBride-Chang, C. (1995). What is phonological awareness? *Journal of Educational Psychology, 87,* 179–192.

McDaniel, C. E., Watson, T. S., Freeland, J. T., Smith, S. L., Jackson, B., & Skinner, C. H. (2001, May). *Comparing silent repeated reading and teacher previewing using silent reading comprehension rate.* Paper presented at the Annual Convention of the Association for Applied Behavior Analysis, New Orleans.

McDougal, J. L., Clonan, S. M., & Martens, B. K. (2000). Using organized change procedures to promote the acceptability of prereferral intervention services: The school-based intervention team project. *School Psychology Quarterly, 15,* 149–171.

McLean, M., Bryant, P., & Bradley, L. (1987). Rhymes, nursery rhymes, and reading in early childhood. *Merrill–Palmer Quarterly, 33,* 255–281.

Messick, S. (1995). Validity of psychological assessment: Validation of inferences from persons' responses and performance as scientific inquiry into score meaning. *American Psychologist, 50,* 741–749.

Methe, S. A., & Hintze, J. M. (2003). Evaluating teacher modeling as a strategy to increase student reading behavior. *School Psychology Review, 32,* 617–623.

Miller, W. H. (1982). *Reading correction kit* (2nd ed.). New York: Center of Applied Research in Education.

Myerson, J., & Hale, S. (1984). Practical implications of the matching law. *Journal of Applied Behavior Analysis, 17,* 367–380.

National Center for Educational Statistics. (2003). *National assessment of educational progress.* (Available online at *http://www.nces.ed.gov/*)

National Reading Panel. (2000). *Teaching children to read: An evidence-based assessment of the scientific research literature on reading and its implications for reading instruction* (Available online at *http //www.nichd.nih.gov/publications/nrp/smallbook.htm*)

National Research Council. (1998). *Preventing reading difficulties in young children.* Washington, DC: National Academy Press.

Nelson, J. R., Smith, D. J., & Dodd, J. M. (1992). The effects of a summary skills strategy to students identified as learning disabled on their comprehension of science text. *Education and Treatment of Children, 15,* 228–243.

Newby, R. F., Caldwell, J., & Recht, D. R. (1989). Improving the reading comprehension of children with dysphonetic and dyseidetic dyslexia using story grammar. *Journal of Learning Disabilities, 22,* 373–380.

Notari-Syverson, A., O'Connor, R. E., & Vadasy, P. F. (1998). *Ladders to literacy: A preschool activity book.* Baltimore: Brookes.

O'Connor, R. E., Notari-Syverson, A., & Vadasy, P. F. (1998). *Ladders to literacy: A kindergarten activity book.* Baltimore: Brookes.

Open Court. (1995). *Collections for young scholars.* Worthington, OH: Author.

O'Shea, L. J., Munson, S. M., & O'Shea, D. J. (1984). Error correction in oral reading: Evaluating the effectiveness of three procedures. *Education and Treatment of Children, 7,* 203–214.

Otis-Wilborn, A. K. (1984). *The evaluation of the effects of four reading instructional procedures on the achievement of hearing-impaired children.* Unpublished doctoral dissertation, University of Kansas, Lawrence.

Pany, D., Jenkins, J. R., & Schreck, J. (1982). Vocabulary instruction: Effects on word knowledge and reading comprehension. *Learning Disability Quarterly, 5,* 202–215.

Parker, S. M., Quigely, M. C., & Reilly, J. B. (1999). *Improving student reading comprehension through the use of literacy circles*. Master's research project, Saint Xavier University, Chicago, IL (ERIC Document Reproduction Service No. ED433504).

Pearson, P. D., & Johnson, D. D. (1978). *Teaching reading comprehension*. New York: Holt, Rinehart & Winston.

Perfetti, C. (1977). Language comprehension and fast decoding: Some psycholinguistic prerequisites for skilled reading comprehension. In J. Guthrie (Ed.), *Cognition, curriculum, and comprehension* (pp. 20–41). Newark, DE: International Reading Association.

Popkin, J., & Skinner, C. H. (2003). Enhancing academic performance in a classroom serving students with serious emotional disturbance: Interdependent group contingencies with randomly selected components. *School Psychology Review, 32*, 282–295.

Pratt, A. C., & Brady, S. (1988). Relation of phonological awareness to reading disability in children and adults. *Journal of Educational Psychology, 80*, 319–323.

Raphael, T. (1986). Teaching question/answer relationship, revisited. *Reading Teacher, 39*, 516–522.

Rashotte, C.A., & Torgesen, J. K. (1985). Repeated reading and reading fluency in learning disabled children. *Reading Research Quarterly, 20*, 180–188.

Renaissance Learning. (2002). *Accelerated reading: Learning information system for reading and literacy systems*. Wisconsin Rapids, WI: Author.

Robinson, D. H., & Skinner, C. H. (1996). Why graphic organizers facilitate search processes: Fewer words of efficient indexing? *Contemporary Educational Psychology, 21*, 166–180.

Robinson, F. P. (1946). *Effective study*. New York: Harper.

Rose, T. L. (1984a). The effects of two pre-preparative procedures on oral reading. *Journal of Learning Disabilities, 17*, 544–548.

Rose, T. L. (1984b). The effects of previewing on retarded learners' oral reading. *Education and Training of the Mentally Retarded, 17*, 49–53.

Rose, T. L. (1984c). Effects of previewing on oral reading of mainstreamed behaviorally disordered students. *Behavioral Disorders, 10*, 33–39.

Rosenshine, B. V. (1980). How time is spent in elementary classrooms. In C. Denham & A. Lieberman (Eds.), *Time to learn* (pp. 107–126). Washington, DC: U.S. Department of Education.

Rosner, J. (1975). *Helping children overcome learning difficulties*. New York: Walker.

Rousseau, M. K., & Yung Tam, B. K. (1991). The efficacy of previewing and discussion of key words on the oral reading proficiency of bilingual learners with speech and language impairments. *Education and Treatment of Children, 14*, 199–209.

Samuels, S. J. (1979). The method of repeated readings. *Reading Teacher, 32*, 403–408.

Samuels, S. J. (1987). Information processing abilities and reading. *Journal of Learning Disabilities, 20*, 18–22.

Schumaker, J., Deshler, D., Alley, G., Warner, M., & Denton, P. (1982). Multipass: A learning strategy for improving reading comprehension. *Learning Disability Quarterly, 5*, 295–304.

Shapiro, E. S. (2004a). *Academic skills problems: Direct assessment and intervention* (3rd ed.). New York: Guilford Press.

Shapiro, E. S. (2004b). *Academic skills problems workbook* (rev. ed.). New York: Guilford Press.

Sharp, S., & Skinner, C. H. (in press). Using interdependent group contingencies with randomly selected criteria and paired reading to enhance class-wide reading performance. *Journal of Applied School Psychology*.

Shinn, M. R. (Ed.). (1989). *Curriculum-based measurement: Assessing special children*. New York: Guilford Press.

Shinn, M. R. (Ed.). (1998). *Advanced applications of curriculum-based measurement*. New York: Guilford Press.

Shinn, M. R., Good, R. H., III, Knutson, N., & Tilly, W. D., III (1992). Curriculum-based measurement of oral reading fluency: A confirmatory analysis of its relation to reading. *School Psychology Review, 21*, 459–479.

Shinn, M. R., & Hubbard, D. (1992). Curriculum-based measurement and problem-solving assessment: Basic procedures and outcomes. *Focus on Exceptional Children, 24*, 1–20.

Sindelar, P. T., Monda, L. E., & O'Shea, L. J. (1990). Effects of repeated readings on instructional- and mastery-level readers. *Journal of Educational Research, 83*, 220–226.

Skinner, C. H. (1998). Preventing academic skills deficits. In T. S. Watson & F. M. Gresham (Eds.), *Handbook of child behavior therapy* (pp. 61–82). New York: Plenum Press.

Skinner, C. H. (2002). An empirical analysis of interspersal research: Evidence, implications and applications of the discrete task completion hypothesis. *Journal of School Psychology, 40*, 347–368.

Skinner, C. H., Adamson, K. L., Woodward, J. R., Jackson, R. R., Atchison, L. A., & Mims, J. W. (1993). The effects of models' rates of reading on students' reading during listening previewing. *Journal of Learning Disabilities, 26*, 674–681.

Skinner, C. H., Cooper, L., & Cole, C. L. (1997). The effects of oral presentation previewing rates on reading performance. *Journal of Applied Behavior Analysis, 30*, 331–333.

Skinner, C. H., Logan, P., Robinson, D. H., Robinson, S. L. (1997). Myths and realities of modeling as a reading intervention: Beyond acquisition. *School Psychology Review, 26*, 437–447.

Skinner, C. H., Neddenriep, C. E., Bradley-Klug, K. L., & Ziemann, J. M. (2002). Advances in curriculum-based measurement: Alternative rate measures for assessing reading skills in pre- and advanced readers. *Behavior Analyst Today, 3*, 270–281.

Skinner, C. H., & Shapiro, E. S. (1989). A comparison of taped-words and drill interventions on reading fluency in adolescents with behavior disorders. *Education and Treatment of Children, 12*, 123–133.

Skinner, C. H., Skinner, A. L., & Armstrong, K. (2000). Shaping leisure reading persistence in a client with chronic schizophrenia. *Psychiatric Rehabilitation Journal, 24*, 52–57.

Skrtic, T. M. (1991). *Behind special education: A critical analysis of professional culture and school organization*. Denver, CO: Love Publishing.

Smith, S. B., Simmons, D. C., & Kame'enui, E. J. (1995). *Synthesis of research on phonological awareness: Principles and implications for reading acquisition*. (Available online at *http://idea.uoregon.edu/~ncite/documents/techrep/tech21.html*)

Sorrell, A. L. (1990). Three reading comprehension strategies: TELLS, story mapping, and QARs. *Academic Therapy, 25*, 359–368.

Spargo, E. (1989a). *Timed readings* (3rd ed.). Providence, RI: Jamestown Publishers.

Spargo, E. (1989b). *Timed readings in literature level* (3rd ed.). Providence, RI: Jamestown Publishers.

Speece, D.L., & Case, L. P. (2001). Classification in context: An alternative approach to identifying early reading disability. *Journal of Educational Psychology, 93*, 735–749.

Stahl, S. A., Duffy-Hester, A. M., & Stahl, K. A. (1998). Everything you wanted to know about phonics (but were afraid to ask). *Reading Research Quarterly, 33*, 338–355.

Stahl, S. A., & Murray, B. A. (1994). Defining phonological awareness and its relationship to early reading. *Journal of Educational Psychology, 86*, 221–234.

Stanovich, K. E. (1986). Matthew effects in reading: Some consequences of individual differences in the acquisition of reading. *Reading Research Quarterly, 21*, 360–406.

Stein, M., Johnson, B., & Gutlohn, L. (1999). Analyzing beginning reading programs: The relationship between decoding instruction and text. *Remedial and Special Education, 20*, 275–287.

Torgesen, J. K., Alexander, A. W., Wagner, R. K., Rashotte, C. A., Voeller, K. S., & Conway, T. (2001). Intensive remedial instruction for children with severe reading disabilities: Immediate and long-term outcomes from two instructional approaches. *Journal of Learning Disabilities, 34,* 33–58.

Torgesen, J. K., & Bryant, B. R. (1994a). *Test of phonological awareness.* Austin, TX: PRO-ED.

Torgesen, J. K. & Bryant, B. R. (1994b). *Phonological awareness training for reading.* Austin, TX: PRO-ED.

Torgesen, J. K., Wagner, R. K., & Rashotte, C. A. (1994). Longitudinal studies of phonological processing and reading. *Journal of Learning Disabilities, 27*, 276–287.

Tunmer, W. E., Herriman, M. L., & Nesdale, A. R. (1988). Metalinguistic abilities and beginning reading. *Reading Research Quarterly, 23*, 134–158.

U.S. Department of Education. (1999). *Reading Excellence Program Overview.* (Available online at *http://www.ed.gov/offices/OESE/REA/overview.html*)

U.S. Department of Education. (2004). *Proven methods: Reading.* (Available online at *http://www.ed.gov/nclb/methods/reading/edpicks.jhtml?src=rt*)

Vargas, J. S. (1984). What are your exercises teaching? An analysis of stimulus control in instructional materials. In W. L. Heward, T. E. Heron, D. S. Hill, & J. Trap-Porter (Eds.), *Focus on behavior analysis in education* (pp. 126–141). Columbus, OH: Merrill.

Vaughn, S., Linan-Thompson, S., & Hickman, P. (2003). Response to instruction as a means of identifying students with reading/learning disabilities. *Exceptional Children, 69*, 391–409.

Vellutino, F. R., Scanlon, D. M., & Tanzman, M. S. (1998). The case for early intervention in diagnosing specific reading disability. *Journal of School Psychology, 36*, 367–397.

Wagner, R., Torgesen, J., & Rashotte, C. (1999). *Comprehensive test of phonological processing.* Austin, TX: PRO-ED.

Wallace, M. A., Cox, E. A., & Skinner, C. H. (2003). Increasing independent seat-work: Breaking large assignments into smaller assignments and teaching a student with retardation to recruit reinforcement. *School Psychology Review, 23*, 132–142.

Walsh, D. J., Price, G. G., & Gillingham, M. G. (1988). The critical but transitory importance of letter naming. *Reading Research Quarterly, 23*, 108–122.

Wolery, M., Bailey, D. B., Jr., & Sugai, G. M. (1988). *Effective teaching: Principles and procedures of applied behavior analysis with exceptional children.* Boston: Allyn & Bacon.

Wong, B. Y. L. (1986). Problems and issues in the definition of learning disabilities. In J. K. Torgesen & B. Y. L. Wong (Eds.), *Psychological and Educational Perspectives on Learning Disabilities* (pp. 1–26). New York: Academic Press.

Worden, P. E., & Boettcher, W. (1990). Young children's acquisition of alphabet knowledge. *Journal of Reading Behavior, 22*, 277–295.

Ysseldyke, J., & Christenson, S. (1993). *The instructional environment system—II.* Longmont, CO: Sopris West.

Index

"f" following a page number indicates a figure; "t" following a page number indicates a table.